# KEYS TO
# MEDICATIONS AND
# DRUG INTERACTIONS

## Marcy Portnoff Gever, R.Ph., M.Ed.
### Pharmacist/Patient Education Specialist

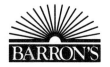

BARRON'S

The information in this book is intended to provide general information about medications and is not intended for personal advice. If you have a specific question about a medication or drug interaction, please ask your doctor or pharmacist. The publisher and author disclaim any personal liability for advice or information presented herein.

*All inquiries should be addressed to:*
Barron's Educational Series, Inc.
250 Wireless Boulevard
Hauppauge, New York 11788

Library of Congress Catalog Card No. 91-20597
International Standard Book No. 0-8120-4749-4

**Library of Congress Cataloging-in-Publication Data**
Gever, Marcy Portnoff.
  Keys to medications and drug interactions / Marcy Portnoff Gever.
        p.   cm. — (Barron's retirement keys)
  Includes index.
  ISBN 0-8120-4749-4
  1. Drug interactions—Popular works.    2. Geriatric pharmacology—
Popular works.    I. Title.   II. Series.
RM302.G48        1991
615'.7045—dc20
91-20597
CIP

PRINTED IN THE UNITED STATES OF AMERICA
2345    5500    987654321

To Eric and Stacy
and
to my husband, Larry N. Gever, Pharm. D.,
for his review of the manuscript
and, most of all, for his encouragement


A special thank you to my family for their insightful comments:
Gloria and Sid Shanken
Rosalind Gever
Harold Gever, M.D.
Camille and Jerry Portnoff

# CONTENTS

# INTRODUCTION

You may read any Key in this book out of sequence; however, you will have a much better understanding of the way your medications interact if you read Part I first. To find your medication, you may look for its name in the index, or you may go directly to the Key that discusses the drug category (for example, anticoagulants) to which your medication belongs.

Each key dealing with specific drugs provides background information about the medical condition or the classification of medication to be discussed. Most Keys provide two more sections, "The Medications" and "Side Effects and Drug Interactions."

At the end of each Key in Parts II–IV is a drug interaction chart that provides the following information:

1. Identification of the medications that interact.
2. A drug interaction rating that describes the potential degree of harm, and the frequency with which the interaction tends to occur.
3. The expected effect or outcome of the interaction.
4. Action that may be taken to avoid the interaction or to minimize any side effects that may occur.

Drugs that interact are indicated by name in the chart, as Drug A/Drug B. Drug A will always be the medication discussed in that particular Key. Drug B is discussed in another Key.

The result of the interaction will be located in the Key for the drug that is affected. For example, if you want to check on the interaction between digoxin and Questran, you may check either Key 17 (Digoxin) or Key 18 (Medications That Reduce Cholesterol). However, you will find the result of this interaction in the Key that discusses digoxin because it is the action of digoxin that is disturbed. The action of Questran is not affected.

In many cases, all of the medications in a particular drug category interact in similar manner with other medications. If this is the case, the drug interaction will list the drug category instead of the individual drug. For example, if a medication interacts with all of the beta blockers, the interaction will read "Beta Blockers/Drug B." If the medication interacts with only the beta blocker Inderal, the interaction will be listed as "Inderal/Drug B."

Throughout the Keys, you may notice that the names of some of the medications begin with uppercase letters and others begin with lowercase letters. The reason is that each medication has two names—a brand name and a generic name. A drug name that begins with an uppercase letter represents the brand name of that medication; a drug name that begins with a lowercase letter is the generic name of the medication. For example, Benadryl is the brand name; diphenhydramine, the generic name.

## A Word of Warning

Although this book provides invaluable information about your medications and the drug interactions that may result from various drug combinations, it is not intended as a substitute for good medical care provided by medical professionals. Rather, the purpose of this book is to provide you with information that will help you take a more active patient role by knowing what questions to ask your doctor to enhance your medication treatment and, in the long run, improve your health.

Finally, do not assume that a drug interaction between two drugs will not occur if it is not in this book! Only the drug interactions that are most important to retirees are included in this edition.

# 1

# FACTS AND MYTHS ABOUT DRUG INTERACTIONS

Are you taking more than one medication? If so, you may be aware that one drug can alter the effectiveness or increase the unwanted effects of the other drug when the two are taken together. See how much you know about drug interactions by deciding which of the following statements are FACTS and which are MYTHS.

**FACT OR MYTH 1:** *Drug interactions can be the cause of prolonged illnesses or even fatal reactions to medications.*

**ANSWER:** Fact

Combining some drugs can lead to severe and sometimes unpredictable reactions because the side effects of one or both drugs are enhanced when the drugs are combined. Prolonged illnesses also can be caused by drug interactions in which one drug reduces the effectiveness of another. If you are taking your medications correctly and your illness does not improve, you should tell your doctor. Although there are many reasons why your condition may not improve, drug interactions should always be considered.

**FACT OR MYTH 2:** *Drugs that interact should not be taken on the same day.*

**ANSWER:** Myth

Many times patients *need* to take two drugs that are known to interact. With some medications, the solution is to take the two drugs several hours apart. For example, antacids interact with several drugs by reducing the absorption of these drugs into the bloodstream. Because the drugs are not fully absorbed, they may be less effective. This drug interaction can be minimized by taking the antacid 2 hours before or after the other medication.

If you must take two medications that interact, and the interaction cannot be eliminated by separating the doses, your doctor will probably want to see you regularly. It is extremely important that you keep your appointments so that the doctor can check for signs of either drug toxicity or (the other extreme) lack of effectiveness.

**FACT OR MYTH 3:** *Drug interactions tend to be more frequent and more severe in people over age 50.*

**ANSWER:** Fact

There are two reasons why people over the age of 50 are more likely to experience side effects caused by drug interactions. First, underlying conditions such as diabetes, hypertension, and kidney impairment become more common with advancing age. People who have these underlying conditions are generally more sensitive to drug side effects. Second, older people tend to have more illnesses than younger people and tend to take more medications simultaneously. As the number of drugs increases, so does the potential risk for drug interactions.

**FACT OR MYTH 4:** *If you discover that you are taking two drugs that interact, you should stop one of the drugs immediately.*

**ANSWER:** Myth

Unless you are experiencing an adverse reaction from the drugs, you should not stop taking either drug without speaking to your doctor first. There are two reasons. First, some drugs, such as beta blockers, should not be stopped abruptly. Doing so may evoke a severe adverse reaction (for example, angina or heart attack in the case of beta blockers). Second, people react differently to medications, especially when the medications are combined. For this reason one person may be able to safely take both drugs at the same time, whereas another person could become very ill. This explains why your doctor must keep a close watch on your drug therapy.

**FACT OR MYTH 5:** *Interactions involving nonprescription drug products are not as dangerous as interactions involving prescription drugs.*

**ANSWER:** Myth

Nonprescription medications are not innocuous. In fact, the combination of some nonprescription drug products with prescription medications may be potentially more dangerous than most people realize. Because many people do not think that nonprescription drugs can be harmful, they fail to check with their pharmacist or doctor for possible drug interactions. Many of the drugs available today without a prescription were once prescription drugs. Although they can now be purchased over the counter, their side effects and their potential to interact with other drugs (including alcohol) still exist. If you plan to take a combination of nonprescription drug products, it is a good idea to make sure they do not interact by checking with your pharmacist.

**FACT OR MYTH 6:** *Foods that may interact with your medication should be eliminated from your diet.*

**ANSWER:** Myth

You may have seen a label on your prescription bottle that reads "Do not take this medication with milk or dairy products." Some patients have interpreted this to mean that they could not drink milk or eat cheese for several days, until their drug treatment was completed. However, there is no need to eliminate dairy products from your diet if you take the medication at least 1 hour before or 2 hours after ingesting these products. Ask your pharmacist to explain any cautionary label to be sure you understand exactly what is meant.

# 2

# AFTER YOU SWALLOW A MEDICATION

After being swallowed and traveling past the throat, the medication travels through the esophagus and drops into the stomach. Once there, stomach acid causes the medication to disintegrate into small pieces that can dissolve in the intestinal fluid. Only dissolved medicine can later be absorbed into the bloodstream.

## The Journey in the Bloodstream

The dissolved medication moves down the intestinal tract from the stomach to the small intestine and through the wall of the intestine into the bloodstream. Once in the bloodstream, the medication takes one of the following routes:

1. It may travel directly to its receptor site (a specific area in the body that the drug acts upon).
2. Alternatively, it may go directly to the liver, where it may be metabolized (changed) into other chemical forms that may or may not have the same medication action as the original drug. The drug then travels to its receptor site to produce its action.

After completing its action, the medication leaves its receptor site and travels to the liver or kidneys to be eliminated from the body. If the drug goes to the kidneys, it may be eliminated in the urine. However, if it goes to the liver, it may be (a) eliminated in the stool, or (b) metabolized again, this time into a form that is readily eliminated in the urine or the stool.

Some medications, such as antacids and laxatives, are not absorbed in the bloodstream because they act directly on the walls of the intestinal tract. When these medications complete their action, they are eliminated in the stool.

## A Medication Traffic Jam

A drug interaction may occur during any phase of the medication's journey. If one medication interferes with another medication's absorption into the bloodstream, the way it is metabolized, the way it circulates in the bloodstream, its action at the receptor site, or the way it is eliminated from the body, the action of the second medication may be less effective or it may produce unwanted side effects.

# 3

## THE MEDICATION DOSAGE THAT IS RIGHT FOR YOU

How do you know what the right *medication dosage* is for you? This is really a job for your doctor, but your input can make a difference in your drug treatment. For example, if you need a medication for pain, your doctor may choose from a wide variety of pain medications that are available on the market. In deciding which drug is the best for you, your doctor may consider some of these questions:

1. How severe is the pain—mild, moderate or severe?
2. How old is the patient, and how much does she weigh?
3. Is the patient allergic to codeine? Does she have an ulcer condition?
4. Does the patient have to drive a car, go to work, or do tasks that require alertness?
5. How long will the patient be using the pain reliever—a week, or several months or years?
6. Is the patient taking other medications that cannot be combined safely with certain pain relievers?

On the basis of these considerations and perhaps others as well, your doctor will choose the best possible pain reliever and dosage for you. However, you can help your doctor decide which pain reliever is best for you by providing an accurate history of your previous illnesses, information about any medication allergies, and a list of the medications you are currently taking. When you have begun taking the drug, you can help your doctor determine if the prescribed dosage is right for you by contacting him if you experience medication side effects or if the medication isn't working. In most cases a simple dosage adjustment will solve the problem, but sometimes your doctor may decide to change the medication.

The fact is that getting the right dosage for some medications is very tricky and may require "fine tuning." Your doctor may want to examine the concentration of the drug in your blood, referred to as the "blood level," to make sure that the drug concentration from the dosage you take is within a certain range. If the blood level of a drug is too high, you may begin to experience medication side effects. If the blood level is too low, the drug may be less effective. Taking blood samples periodically to examine the medication blood level is a useful check—this is why it is important that you keep appointments for blood work. More often than not, though, drug blood levels are not necessary. Your doctor can usually assess the effectiveness of drug therapy by measuring indicators of your condition. For example, to see whether your blood pressure medication is effective, your doctor will simply take your blood pressure.

There are four things you *should not do* during your medication therapy:

1. Do not skip doses or stop taking the medication unless your doctor tells you to do so—skipping doses can be dangerous with some medications.

2. Do not double the dosage because you think the medication is not working—some drugs take a long time to act.

3. Do not change the dosage in any way without your doctor's approval. (As a pharmacist, I was surprised to learn that one of my patients had decided to cut the dosage of his heart medication by half because "the drug was too expensive"!)

4. Do not take nonprescription drug products with a new medication until you check for possible drug interactions with your doctor or pharmacist.

When you get your prescription filled, ask your pharmacist to tell you the best way to take the medication.

# 4

# WHAT IS A DRUG INTERACTION?

A *drug interaction* is the result of two or more medications interfering with each other. Although most medications can be taken together safely, many may become more potent or, alternatively, lose their effectiveness when combined with other drugs.

Some medications, when taken with others, can cause unexpected side effects that would normally not occur if either drug were taken alone. A good example is the drug interaction between Flagyl (an antibiotic) and terpin hydrate (a non-prescription cough expectorant). When taken together, these two medications can cause severe nausea, vomiting, throbbing headaches, flushing of the face, and palpitations.

Most people would not expect an antibiotic and a cough medicine to produce such serious side effects, especially when they've taken antibiotics with cough medicines that were prescribed for them by their doctors. So why does this interaction occur? There are two reasons. First, Flagyl is one of the few antibiotics that interacts adversely with alcohol. Second, terpin hydrate contains a large amount of alcohol (42%). The drug interaction is caused by Flagyl's interference with the metabolism (breakdown) of alcohol in the bloodstream.

Does this mean that Flagyl cannot be combined with cough medicines? No, several cough products that do not contain alcohol are available, and these can be taken safely with Flagyl.

# 5

## HOW DRUG INTERACTIONS CAN AFFECT YOUR TREATMENT

Combining one medication with other medications may be a real art...and nonprescription drug products are no exception. The following story illustrates how two apparently "harmless" medications (one a prescription drug; the other a nonprescription drug) produced an unexpected reaction in one retiree:

A 62-year-old woman and her 66-year-old husband boarded a luxury liner. It was the woman's first cruise, in celebration of her husband's long awaited retirement. To prevent motion sickness, her doctor prescribed Transderm Scōp, a medication enclosed in a round bandagelike patch, which is placed behind the ear.

On the day of departure, the woman did everything right—she unwrapped the patch and applied it behind her ear approximately 4 hours before boarding. Shortly after boarding, suddenly and without warning, she began to feel lightheaded, dizzy, and drowsy. She complained of a dry mouth and her vision was slightly blurred.

Although these side effects can occur with the use of Transderm Scōp alone, the ship's doctor could not understand why the woman's reaction to the drug was so severe—until she told him that she had taken another medication, Chlor-Trimeton, 1 hour earlier. Like most antihistamines, Chlor-Trimeton can also cause dizziness, drowsiness, and the other side effects listed above, especially in people over age 50.

Combined, these two drugs produced a severe reaction in this woman. However, her experience does not mean that you would react in the same way. As stated in Key 1, people react differently to medications and to combinations of medications. For example, if you do not usually feel drowsy when you take an antihistmine, your doctor might allow you to combine it with Transderm Scōp.

The example above illustrates how two medications that have similar side effects can cause a serious reaction when they are combined. Here are three other ways that drug interactions can affect your treatment:

1. One medication may become more potent when it is combined with another medication. If it becomes too potent, you may experience side effects. One drug may prevent another from being eliminated from the body, thereby increasing its potency (if the drug is not eliminated, it continues to act).

2. One medication may become less effective when it is combined with another medication. If it loses too much of its effectiveness, your medical condition may worsen.

3. Two medications used for different medical conditions may be similar in chemical structure and, when combined, may produce more potent action, with increased risk of side effects. Some drugs are similar to each other in their action, but are used for different purposes. Example: Chlor-Trimeton for allergy and diphenhyramine in over-the-counter sleep aids. Both are antihistamines and when combined, may cause severe dry mouth, blurred vision, and the like. In item 1 above, one drug is disturbing the other's action. In this case, the action of neither drug is disturbed, but both have the same action and side effects. When combined, the drug's action may be more potent and side effects more pronounced (like an overdose).

Finally, keep in mind that nonprescription drug products *can* and *do* interact, even with other nonprescription drugs!

10

# 6

# TEN WAYS THAT DRUGS
# MAY INTERACT

The ways that medications can interfere with each other are numerous! Moreover, drug interactions may occur in different areas in the body—in the intestinal tract; in the blood; at the receptor site; in the liver, where some drugs are metabolized (broken down); and in the kidneys, where some drugs are eliminated from the body.

Here are ten examples of the ways in which drugs may interact with each other:

1. *Decreased absorption.* One drug may alter the absorption of another drug. If a drug is not completely absorbed into the bloodstream, it may be less effective. Conversely, if it is absorbed more extensively than is normal into the bloodstream, it may have a too potent and perhaps dangerous effect.

2. *Interference with blood proteins* ("protein binding"). Medications travel through the bloodstream to reach the areas in the body where they produce their actions. Along the way, some drugs attach themselves to proteins that are also circulating in the bloodstream. Once attached to a protein, the drug is unable to act—it is in an "inactive" state. The amount of a medication that binds to these proteins is different for each drug. Some drugs, like Coumadin, bind excessively with the proteins; other drugs do not bind at all.

   Drug interactions occur when two drugs that want to bind with proteins are circulating in the bloodstream. In that case one drug may be bound to a protein, and another drug (with more "binding power") may dislodge the first drug and take its place on the protein. If too much drug

11

is dislodged, it is "free" to cause problems. In effect, there is a tug-of-war between drugs for the limited number of proteins circulating in the blood.

3. *Drug "antagonism."* Two drugs may oppose each other's action.

4. *Blocking at the receptor site.* One drug may interfere with the action of another drug at its receptor site (the area in the body where the drug produces its action).

5. *Increased drug metabolism.* One drug may increase the metabolism (break-down) of another drug into its inactive form; the result may be to reduce the affected drug's overall effectiveness.

6. *Decreased drug metabolism.* One drug may decrease the metabolism of another drug into its inactive form; the result may be to increase the affected drug's potency.

7. *Inhibited drug elimination.* One drug may prevent another drug from being eliminated from the body. If the drug is not eliminated, it will remain in the bloodstream and continue to produce its action, resulting in a more potent and possibly dangerous effect.

8. *Duplication of side effects: different drug classes.* Two medications may have similar side effects. When the drugs are combined, side effects are more likely to occur and may be more intense than if either drug were used alone.

9. *Duplication of side effects: same drug class.* Two medications may be in the same drug classification. If both drugs are taken together, side effects common to both drugs are likely to occur.

10. *Drug duplication.* Two drug products may contain the same active ingredient. When both products are taken, the double dose of the active ingredient can lead to an overdose.

# 7

## SCHEDULING MEDICATIONS TO PREVENT DRUG INTERACTIONS

A woman in her middle 50's stopped by my pharmacy counter. As I greeted her, she spoke softly. "I don't know if I should tell you this—it's really terrible, but I couldn't help it!" What could she have done? Did she take an overdose of something?

"I'm taking tetracycline," she began, "and my doctor told me not to take it with dairy products. But something came over me—I just had to have an ice cream sundae! Will the tetracycline still work?"

I sighed with relief. "Don't be upset," I began, "you didn't do anything wrong. When did you start taking the antibiotic?"

"Five days ago," she replied, "and until today I didn't cheat—no dairy products for five days."

"Oh, no! Didn't anybody explain to you that you could still eat dairy products during your therapy, but not within one hour of taking your medication?"

She looked bewildered. "No. I thought that I had to avoid milk, cheese, yogurt, and ice cream for ten days."

Unfortunately, misunderstandings like this one tend to occur more often than they should. There are many examples of drug interactions in which one drug alters the absorption of another drug. Food may also alter the absorption of some drugs, thereby reducing their effectiveness. To avoid this type of drug interaction, you may simply take one medication one to two hours before or after the other medication (or food). This way, the two drugs won't mix in the intestinal tract. Drug interactions of this type occur most frequently with antacids or food, which prevent or reduce the absorption of some drugs into the bloodstream.

On the other hand, some drug interactions cannot be avoided by separating the drug doses by one or two hours. For example, if you are taking medication for high blood pressure and also need a nonprescription medication for congested sinuses, you cannot use a decongestant, even four hours after you've taken your blood pressure medication. For this kind of drug interaction, you must avoid one of the medications (in this case, the decongestant) unless your doctor tells you otherwise.

Combining prescription medications and nonprescription drug products can be tricky because your doctor doesn't know which over-the-counter drug products you are selecting. In addition, many nonprescription drug products contain several active ingredients, any one of which may interact with your prescription medication. It is a good idea, therefore, to check with your pharmacist or doctor for possible drug interactions before you take any nonprescription drug product.

# 8

## COMBINING SOME DRUGS CAN BENEFIT YOU

Have you ever heard of a "good" drug interaction? Just the term "drug interaction" itself conjures up a feeling of danger. Questions such as "If I take these two medications together, will I still be alive tomorrow morning to talk about it?" loom in the back of our minds.

Actually, a drug interaction is nothing more than two medications interfering with each other. The results may be bad or (less often) good. As you may have guessed, there are a lot more bad interactions than good ones. However, taking a combination of two medicines is sometimes more effective and produces fewer side effects than taking larger doses of either medicine alone.

Here is an example of a "beneficial" drug interaction between *Apresoline and Inderal.* Apresoline, a blood pressure medication, causes an increased heart rate in some people. When this happens, a beta blocker such as Inderal may be added to the drug therapy. This combination is desirable for two reasons: First, beta blockers act by reducing the heart rate, thereby counteracting the increase caused by Apresoline. Second, they too lower blood pressure. Because both drugs reduce blood pressure, less of each drug is needed to achieve the desired effect. For most drugs, the risk of side effects increases when the dosage increases. Therefore, reducing the dosage of each medicine also reduces the risk of side effects.

# 9

# THE DRUG INTERACTION RATING SYSTEM

What are the chances that an *interaction* between two of your medications will cause you to experience side effects? This is the million-dollar question...because nobody, not even your doctor, can predict whether you will be the one to have a bad reaction to a particular drug combination. Every person is different and may react differently to each medication and to each combination of medications.

Reports and studies of drug interactions help us to predict how frequently a drug interaction between two drugs may occur, and what percentage of the population may react to a particular combination of drugs. These studies also help us to predict how harmful a drug interaction is likely to be. There is, however, no way to predict how you personally will react.

To determine how important a drug interaction may be, each interaction has been given a rating based on two factors:

1. the frequency with which the interaction may occur and
2. the degree of harm that may be caused by the interaction.

## Frequency of Drug Interactions Causing Side Effects

Drug interactions that occur frequently are rated either "A" (if more harmful) or "C" (if less harmful). These are the drug interactions that affect most people, such as the interaction between barbiturates and alcohol. Drug interactions that are less frequent are rated "B" (if more harmful) or "D" (if less harmful).

## Degree of Harm That May be Caused by Drug Interactions

Drug interactions may be harmful in two ways. The first, obvious way is by producing side effects; the second way is by reducing the effectiveness of one or both of the drugs taken.

Drug interactions that are "more harmful" are rated "A" (if occurring frequently) or "B" (if occurring less frequently). They are the kind that are more likely to cause either (a) severe side effects, or (b) a worsening of the medical condition because the medication has become less effective or even completely ineffective.

Drug interactions that are "less harmful" are rated "C" (if occurring frequently) or "D" (if occurring less frequently). These kinds of interactions (such as a dry mouth or reduced effectiveness of a pain reliever) tend to be bothersome, but usually do not cause great harm to most people. (This does not mean that a C- or D-rated interaction cannot harm you; great harm, however, is less likely to occur.)

## The Drug Interaction Rating System

The drug interaction rating system may be summarized as follows:

"A" indicates a drug interaction that may cause serious harm and occurs frequently.

"B" indicates a drug interaction that may cause serious harm but occurs less frequently.

"C" indicates a drug interaction that is less harmful but occurs frequently.

"D" indicates a drug interaction that is less harmful and occurs less frequently.

# 10

## ULCER MEDICATIONS

*Peptic ulcers* may be described as inflamed, craterlike lesions that form in the lining of the gastrointestinal tract. They are painful and usually occur repeatedly. Since peptic ulcers are aggravated by stomach acid, the amount of stomach acid that comes in contact with the ulcer must be minimized if the ulcer is to heal.

### The Medications

Three categories of medications prescribed to treat peptic ulcers include those that:
1. reduce the amount of acid secreted in the stomach: *Axid, Pepcid, Tagamet,* and *Zantac.*
2. provide a protective coating to the ulcer to shield the ulcer from the acid: *Carafate.*
3. neutralize the acid present in the gastrointestinal tract: antacids such as *Maalox* or *Mylanta.*

Your ulcer treatment may involve one, two, or all of these categories.

### Side Effects and Drug Interactions

#### Axid, Pepcid, Tagamet, and Zantac

These medications interact with many drugs but are rarely affected themselves. Tagamet, for example, retards the metabolism (breakdown) of many other drugs, thereby reducing their elimination from the body. Consequently they may remain in the body and continue to act, resulting in a more potent effect. Tagamet's action, however, remains unchanged.

Some medications, such as the antifungal drug Nizoral, need a lot of acid to dissolve and be absorbed into the bloodstream. Therefore, Nizoral may be less effective if given with any of the drugs that reduce the amount of acid in the intestinal tract.

## Carafate

Carafate may hinder the absorption of other medications, causing them to be less effective. Carafate's action, however, remains unchanged. To minimize this drug interaction, take your other medication two hours before or after Carafate.

## Antacids

Antacids such as Maalox or Mylanta may hinder the absorption of other medications (including Tagamet). Take your other medication two hours before or after the antacid.

### DRUG INTERACTION CHART:
### ULCER MEDICATIONS

| Drug Interaction | Rating* | Potential Effects/Recommendations |
| --- | --- | --- |
| Axid/Aspirin | D | See Key 35. |
| Axid/Nizoral | D | See Key 32. |
| Carafate/Cipro | A | See Key 31. |
| Carafate/Coumadin | D | See Key 19. |
| Carafate/Digoxin | D | See Key 17. |
| Carafate/Dilantin | C | See Key 30. |
| Carafate/Food | A | Carafate has been shown to be more effective when taken on an empty stomach, one to two hours before meals. |
| Carafate/Noroxin | A | See Key 31. |
| Pepcid/Nizoral | D | See Key 32. |
| Tagamet/Alcohol | C | See Key 43. |
| Tagamet/Antacids | D | Tagamet may become less effective. Take the antacid two hours before or after Tagamet. |
| Tagamet/ Benzodiazepines | C | See Key 21. |
| Tagamet/Beta Blockers | A | See Key 14. |
| Tagamet/Cardizem | D | See Key 15. |

| Drug Interaction | Rating* | Potential Effects/Recommendations |
| --- | --- | --- |
| Tagamet/Coumadin | A | See Key 19. |
| Tagamet/Depakene | D | See Key 30. |
| Tagamet/Diabetes Medicines | D | See Key 28. |
| Tagamet/Digoxin | D | See Key 17. |
| Tagamet/Dilantin | A | See Key 30. |
| Tagamet/Iron | D | See Key 41. |
| Tagamet/Narcotic Pain Relievers | B | See Key 26. |
| Tagamet/Nizoral | D | See Key 32. |
| Tagamet/Procardia | A | See Key 15. |
| Tagamet/Procan | A | See Key 16. |
| Tagamet/Quinidine | A | See Key 16. |
| Tagamet/Reglan | D | Tagamet may become less effective. Your doctor may adjust your Tagamet dosage. |
| Tagamet/Tegretol | A | See Key 30. |
| Tagamet/Theophylline | A | See Key 20. |
| Tagamet/TCAs | A | See Key 23. |
| Zantac/Cardizem | D | See Key 15. |
| Zantac/Nizoral | D | See Key 32. |
| Zantac/Procan | B | See Key 16. |

* The rating indicates how harmful a drug interaction may be and how frequently it may occur.

"A" indicates a drug interaction that may cause serious harm and occurs frequently. "B" indicates a drug interaction that may cause serious harm but occurs less frequently. "C" indicates a drug interaction that is less harmful but occurs frequently. "D" indicates a drug interaction that is less harmful and occurs less frequently. See Key 9 for more information about the rating system.

# 11

## GASTROINTESTINAL MEDICATIONS

Spastic colon, pancreatitis, ulcerative colitis, and gastro-esophageal reflux disease (GERD) are only some of the disorders that involve the *gastrointestinal* tract.

### The Medications

There are three categories of gastrointestinal medications:

1. Antispasmodics, which reduce spasms in the intestinal tract, often are prescribed to treat spastic colon, mild ulcerative colitis, and other gastrointestinal conditions that cause diarrhea: *Anaspaz, Banthine, Belladonna, Bentyl, Cantil, Darbid, Daricon, Levsin, Levsinex, Pamine, Pathilon, Pro-Banthine, Quarzan, Robinul* and *Valpin.* Some antispasmodic drug products contain a sedative to reduce stress that may aggravate the condition: *Bellergal-S, Butibel, Donnatal, Kinesed,* and *Librax.*
2. Digestive enzymes prescribed for chronic pancreatitis: *Cotazyme, Pancrease* and *Viokase.*
3. Medications prescribed to treat gastroesophageal reflux disease, a condition that results in repeated heartburn caused by the backward flow of stomach contents into the esophagus: *Reglan* and *Prilosec.*

### Side Effects and Drug Interactions

#### Antispasmodics

The most common side effects of antispasmodics are dry mouth, blurred vision, dizziness, and drowsiness. Other side effects that are infrequent but can be serious are urinary retention (a reduction in the excretion of urine) and higher risk of acute glaucoma (increased pressure in the eyeball).

These side effects are more likely to occur when antispasmodic drugs are taken with other drugs that cause the same kind of side effects, such as antihistamines, phenothiazine-type medications, tricyclic antidepressants, and alcoholic beverages.

### Digestive Enzymes

Cotazyme, Pancrease, or Viokase may lose its effectiveness if taken with some antacids and should therefore be taken at least two hours before or after the antacid.

### Drugs for Gastroesophageal Reflux Disease

Reglan reduces the backward flow of stomach contents into the esophagus by producing contractions in the gastrointestinal tract that push the stomach contents forward into the small intestine. Reglan may also have the same effect on some medications—that is, by pushing the medication into the small intestine, Reglan may interfere with the way some drugs are absorbed into the bloodstream. For example, digoxin, a heart medication, may be less effective, whereas levodopa, a drug for Parkinson's disease, may have a more potent effect when taken with Reglan.

Prilosec may also interfere with the absorption of other drugs.

### DRUG INTERACTION CHART: GASTROINTESTINAL MEDICATIONS

| Drug Interaction | Rating* | Potential Effects/Recommendations |
|---|---|---|
| Antispasmodics/ Antihistamines (not Seldane or Hismanal) | C | You may experience dry mouth, blurred vision, dizziness, and drowsiness. Ask your pharmacist to recommend a cough or cold product that does not contain an antihistamine. |
| Antispasmodics/ Digoxin | B | See Key 17. |
| Antispasmodics/ Levodopa | B | See Key 34. |

| Drug Interaction | Rating* | Potential Effects/Recommendations |
|---|---|---|
| Antispasmodics/ Phenothiazines | B | You may experience dry mouth, blurred vision, and dizziness. Contact your doctor immediately. The dosage of the phenothiazine or the antispasmodic may have to be adjusted. |
| Antispasmodics/TCAs | B | You may experience dry mouth, blurred vision, dizziness, and drowsiness. Tell your doctor immediately. The dosage of the tricyclic medication or the antispasmodic may have to be adjusted. |
| Cotazyme/Antacids | C | Cotazyme may be less effective. Take Cotazyme two hours before or after the antacid. |
| Pancrease/Antacids | C | Pancrease may be less effective. Take Pancrease two hours before or after the antacid. |
| Prilosec/ Benzodiazepines | B | See Key 21. |
| Prilosec/Coumadin | D | See Key 19. |
| Prilosec/Dilantin | B | See Key 30. |
| Reglan/Alcohol | B | See Key 43. |
| Reglan/Antihistamines (not Seldane or Hismanal) | D | You may feel excessively drowsy and dizzy. Ask your pharmacist to recommend a cough or cold product that does not contain an antihistamine. |
| Reglan/Digoxin | B | See Key 17. |
| Reglan/Levodopa | B | See Key 34. |
| Reglan/Narcotic Pain Relievers | D | See Key 26. |
| Reglan/Sandimmune | B | See Key 34. |
| Reglan/Tagamet | D | See Key 10. |
| Viokase/Antacids | C | Viokase may be less effective. Take Viokase two hours before or after the antacid. |

\* The rating indicates how harmful a drug interaction may be and how frequently it may occur.

"A" indicates a drug interaction that may cause serious harm and occurs frequently. "B" indicates a drug interaction that may cause serious harm but occurs less frequently. "C" indicates a drug interaction that is less harmful but occurs frequently. "D" indicates a drug interaction that is less harmful and occurs less frequently. See Key 9 for more information about the rating system.

# 12

## BLOOD PRESSURE MEDICATIONS

*Hypertension* (high blood pressure) is a disease that has no symptoms but can lead to heart attack or stroke. Because of the absence of symptoms, many people do not take their blood pressure medications *consistently*—a practice that may worsen their overall condition.

It is important that you take each dose of your blood pressure medication. Skipping doses or suddenly stopping some blood pressure medications can cause serious side effects, especially if you are taking other medications. Your medications work together to produce their actions—if you skip one medication, the other medication may become either more potent or less effective. Either way, it's a bad scenario.

Blood pressure medications are categorized by the way they act in the body to lower blood pressure. Although used primarily to treat hypertension, some medications are also effective against other conditions, such as angina (heart pain) or water retention. Many factors go into determining which blood pressure medication is right for you. Your doctor will make the choice based on professional judgment.

### The Medications

Listed below are seven categories of medications used to treat high blood pressure. This Key focuses on the three categories of medications prescribed primarily to treat hypertension:

1. angiotensin converting enzyme (ACE) inhibitors: *Capoten, Prinivil* (or *Zestril*), and *Vasotec.*

2. adrenergic blocking agents: *Aldomet, Cardura, Catapres, Hylorel, Hytrin, Ismelin, Minipress, Reserpine, Tenex,* and *Wytensin.*
3. vasodilators: *Apresoline* and *Loniten.*

Four categories of medications are also used for hypertension:
4. diuretics (water pills), discussed in Key 13.
5. beta blockers, discussed in Key 14.
6. heart medications for angina, discussed in Key 15.
7. calcium channel blockers, discussed in Key 15.

Your blood pressure treatment may include more than one medication. Taking two medications together is often more effective (and less likely to cause side effects) than taking a large dose of either medication alone.

## Side Effects and Drug Interactions

### ACE Inhibitors

The ACE inhibitors are sometimes combined with diuretics to produce a stronger effect. However, combining ACE inhibitors and certain diuretics can lead to excess potassium in the blood and to potassium side effects. If you are taking Aldactone, Dyazide, Dyrenium, or Moduretic (or potassium supplements), you should have your potassium blood level checked regularly.

### Adrenergic Blocking Agents

These drugs act by preventing the constriction (closing up) of blood vessels. When the blood vessels are dilated (opened wider), blood pressure is reduced. Adrenergic blocking drugs interact mostly with decongestants, diet aids, and medications used to treat depression—monoamine oxidase inhibitors (MAOIs) and tricyclic antidepressants (TCAs). Decongestants such as Sudafed (pseudoephedrine), ephedrine, and phenylpropanolamine (PPA) can increase blood pressure because they work by constricting blood vessels.

As part of their blood pressure treatment, many people are told by their doctors to lose weight. Ironically, many of the diet aids available without a prescription contain phenylpropanolamine (PPA), an ingredient that suppresses the appetite but can significantly increase blood pressure.

Minipress often produces a reaction that can be serious when you take the *first dose*. You may feel weak, dizzy, and faint. If you have been taking Minipress and are now starting another medication, you may also experience this reaction with the first dose of the new drug. It is a good idea to take these medications for the first time when you're at home and at bedtime. If a bedtime dose is not practicable, remember to sit up or stand up slowly after taking the initial dose to minimize symptoms.

**Vasodilators**

The vasodilators act by relaxing the smooth muscle that surrounds the blood vessels, thereby allowing the blood vessels to dilate (open) to reduce blood pressure. Apresoline may be prescribed with a beta blocker to enhance its effect. (This is a good example of a "beneficial" drug interaction.)

### DRUG INTERACTION CHART:
### BLOOD PRESSURE MEDICATIONS

| Drug Interaction | Rating* | Potential Effects/Recommendations |
|---|---|---|
| ACE Inhibitors/Aspirin | D | The ACE inhibitor may be less effective. If you are taking aspirin for pain (not arthritis), take Tylenol instead. |
| ACE Inhibitors/ Digoxin | D | See Key 17. |
| ACE Inhibitors/ Diuretics | B | If you have been taking Bumex, Edecrin or Lasix for your blood pressure and start an ACE inhibitor, you may feel dizzy or weak approximately two to three hours after the **first dose**. Subsequent doses should not have that effect. |

26

| Drug Interaction | Rating* | Potential Effects/Recommendations |
| --- | --- | --- |
| ACE Inhibitors/ Diuretics (Potassium-Sparing) | B | The amount of potassium in your blood could increase dramatically. If you experience nausea, diarrhea, or muscle weakness, contact your doctor. These symptoms may indicate hyperkalemia (too much potassium). |
| ACE Inhibitors (Capoten)/Food | C | Capoten may be less effective if taken with food. Take Capoten one hour before meals. |
| ACE Inhibitors/ NSAIDs | A | The ACE inhibitor may be less effective. Check your blood pressure regularly. |
| ACE Inhibitors/ Potassium Supplements | B | The amount of potassium in your blood could increase and lead to symptoms of hyperkalemia (too much potassium). If you experience nausea, diarrhea, and muscle weakness, contact your doctor. |
| ACE Inhibitors (Vasotec)/Rifampin | B | Vasotec may be less effective. Check your blood pressure while you are taking rifampin. |
| ACE Inhibitors (Capoten)/Thorazine | B | Dizziness and weakness are possible when you stand up from a lying position. Change your body position slowly. |
| ACE Inhibitors/ Zyloprim | B | Skin rashes, fever, and muscle aches have occurred in some people. Contact your doctor *immediately* if you experience these symptoms. |
| Aldomet/Decongestants | A | Decongestants may increase your blood pressure. Before buying allergy or cough/cold medications, ask your pharmacist whether the medication contains a decongestant. |
| Aldomet/Diabetes Medicines | D | See Key 28. |
| Aldomet/Diet Aids (PPA) | A | Phenylpropanolamine (PPA) may cause your blood pressure to increase. Before you use a diet aid that contains PPA, *consult your doctor*. |

| Drug Interaction | Rating* | Potential Effects/Recommendations |
|---|---|---|
| Aldomet/Haldol | B | See Key 24. |
| Aldomet/Iron | C | Iron may reduce the effectiveness of Aldomet. Take iron two hours before or after Aldomet. |
| Aldomet/Levodopa | D | Both medications may be more potent; this combination is sometimes pre-scribed for patients who are taking levodopa and who need a blood pressure medication. The dosages of both drugs may have to be adjusted. |
| Aldomet/Lithium | B | See Key 24. |
| Aldomet/TCAs | D | Your blood pressure may increase; the tricyclic medication may be less effective. The medication dosages may have to be adjusted. |
| Apresoline/Beta Blockers | C | Both drugs may be more potent; these medications are often combined intentionally to reduce blood pressure. |
| Apresoline/Indocin | B | Apresoline may be less effective. Check your blood pressure regularly. |
| Catapres/Beta Blockers | A | If you miss doses or stop taking Catapres, your blood pressure may increase suddenly. Do not skip doses of either medication. |
| Catapres/TCAs | A | Your blood pressure may increase. If you are being treated for depression, tell your doctor that you are taking Catapres. |
| Ismelin/Decongestants | C | Your blood pressure may increase. In addition, decongestants such as Sudafed or other cold/allergy products that con-tain ephedrine or phenylpropanolamine (PPA) may not be effective. Ask your pharmacist to recommend a cold/allergy product that does not contain a decongestant. |

28

| Drug Interaction | Rating* | Potential Effects/Recommendations |
|---|---|---|
| Ismelin/Diet Aids (PPA) | C | An active ingredient in many diet aids, phenylpropanolamine (PPA) may increase your blood pressure. Also, PPA may be ineffective when taken with Ismelin. Be sure your diet aid does not contain PPA. |
| Ismelin/Haldol (and possibly Ismelin/Hylorel) | D | Ismelin may be less effective, and your blood pressure may increase. Check your blood pressure regularly. |
| Ismelin/Insulin | B | See Key 28. |
| Ismelin/Navane | D | Ismelin may be less effective, and your blood pressure may increase. Check your blood pressure regularly. |
| Ismelin/Thorazine | A | Ismelin may be less effective, and your blood pressure may increase. Check your blood pressure regularly. |
| Ismelin/TCAs | A | Ismelin may be less effective, and your blood pressure may increase. Check your blood pressure regularly. |
| Minipress/Beta Blockers or Minipress/CCBs | A | You may feel dizzy, weak, or faint when you stand up from a lying or sitting position after taking your *first dose* of Minipress. These symptoms may also occur if you are taking Minipress and take the *first dose* of a beta blocker or a calcium channel blocker. These side effects should disappear with the second dose. Move slowly when you change your body position, especially when you sit or stand up. |
| Minipress/NSAIDs | D | Minipress may be less effective when combined with Indocin. Check your blood pressure regularly. |

29

| Drug Interaction | Rating* | Potential Effects/Recommendations |
|---|---|---|
| Reserpine/<br>Decongestants | B | Your blood pressure may increase; the decongestant may be less effective. Ask your pharmacist to recommend a cold/allergy product that does not contain a decongestant. |
| Reserpine/MAOIs | B | Your blood pressure may increase, and you may experience nervousness and insomnia. If you have these symptoms, contact your doctor. |

\* The rating indicates how harmful a drug interaction may be and how frequently it may occur.

"A" indicates a drug interaction that may cause serious harm and occurs frequently. "B" indicates a drug interaction that may cause serious harm but occurs less frequently. "C" indicates a drug interaction that is less harmful but occurs frequently. "D" indicates a drug interaction that is less harmful and occurs less frequently. See Key 9 for more information about the rating system.

# 13

## DIURETICS (WATER PILLS)

*Diuretics*, better known as "water pills," are often pre-scribed to reduce high blood pressure, relieve edema (swelling caused by excess fluid), and treat congestive heart failure (a condition in which the heart muscle has difficulty in pumping the blood through the arteries of the body). One diuretic, Diamox, is sometimes used to treat glaucoma.

### The Medications

The diuretics are divided into categories based on where they work in the kidney to produce their actions. The one thing all diuretics have in common is that they reduce the amount of fluid in the body by increasing urination.

The five diuretic categories are as follows:

1. thiazides: the most common are *chlorothiazide, Diuril, Enduron, Esidrex, hydrochlorothiazide, Hydrodiuril, Renese,* and *Saluron.*
2. thiazide-like diuretics: *chlorthalidone, Diulo, Hygroton, Lozol,* and *Zaroxolyn.*
3. loop diuretics: *Bumex, Edecrin, furosemide,* and *Lasix.*
4. potassium-sparing diuretics: *Aldactone, amiloride, Dyrenium, Midamor, spironalactone,* and *triamterene.*
5. *Diamox* (used mainly for glaucoma).

Some diuretic drug products contain more than one diuretic:

*Aldactazide* = spironalactone and hydrochlorothiazide.
*Dyazide* = triamterene and hydrochlorothiazide.
*Maxide* = triamterene and hydrochlorothiazide.
*Moduretic* = amiloride and hydrochlorothizide.

### Side Effects and Drug Interactions

The most common side effect of diuretics is that they increase urination to the point where you may find yourself

31

heading for the bathroom more frequently than ever before. This can be bothersome if you have to get up several times during the night to empty your bladder. The best way to minimize this problem is to take your diuretic in the morning so that urination will be most frequent during the day. Sometimes, your doctor may specifically prescribe a diuretic for the evening. In this case, follow your doctor's recommendation.

The side effect that you should be most concerned about is a change in your potassium balance. All diuretics can change the amount of potassium in the body, and this change may result in side effects.

1. *Hyperkalemia* (too much potassium in the blood) can lead to side effects involving the heart. Hyperkalemia may be caused by the potassium-sparing diuretics.

2. *Hypokalemia* (not enough potassium in the blood) can lead to weakness, cramping in the legs, and also side effects involving the heart. Hypokalemia may be caused by the potassium-losing diuretics such as the thiazides, thiazide-like diuretics, and loop diuretics.

   If you are taking one of these, your pharmacist has probably labeled your prescription vial with a sticker that reads "Eat a banana or drink 8 ounces of orange juice daily." Bananas and orange juice are two good sources of potassium. Some people, however, need to take an additional potassium supplement to keep enough potassium in their blood.

Potassium balance can be upset further by combining other medications with the diuretic. Therefore, to detect potassium imbalances before they get out of control, your doctor may want to check your *potassium blood level* (the amount of potassium in your blood). Depending on the results of your blood test, your doctor may adjust your diuretic dosage.

Finally, it is important that you keep your appointments for checkups and examinations. Too often, I hear, "Why does my doctor want to see me? I've been taking this medication for two years and will be on it the rest of my life." Beware: your body is changing as you grow older, and you may need a dosage adjustment along the way.

## DRUG INTERACTION CHART: DIURETICS (WATER PILLS)

The term "thiazides" includes the following diuretics: Diulo, Diuril, Enduron, Esidrex, Hydrodiuril, Hygroton, Lozol, Naturetin, Renese, Saluron, and Zaroxolyn.

| Drug Interaction | Rating* | Potential Effects/Recommendations |
|---|---|---|
| Aldactone/Lithium | D | See Key 24. |
| Aldactone/Potassium Supplements | A | The amount of potassium in your blood may become excessive and thereby lead to disturbances in heart function. Your doctor may want to have your potassium blood level checked regularly. |
| Aldactone/Salt Substitutes | B | Most salt substitutes contain large amounts of potassium. If you use *excessive* amounts of salt substitutes, you could absorb too much potassium, which can lead to heart disturbances. |
| Bumex/Lithium | D | See Key 24. |
| Bumex/NSAIDs | C | Bumex may be less effective in lowering your blood pressure. Your doctor may adjust your Bumex dosage or change the pain reliever. |
| Diamox/Aspirin | A | If you are taking large amounts of aspirin (8 regular strength) *every day*, you may experience side effects of Diamox (fatigue, lethargy, confusion, loss of appetite). People who have kidney disease are especially sensitive to this drug interaction. |
| Diamox/Mysoline | B | See Key 22. |
| Diamox/Quinidine | B | See Key 16. |
| Dyrenium or Dyazide/ ACE Inhibitors | D | The amount of potassium in your blood could increase. Your doctor may want you to have your potassium blood level checked regularly. |

| Drug Interaction | Rating* | Potential Effects/Recommendations |
|---|---|---|
| Dyrenium or Dyazide/ Indocin | B | Disturbances in kidney function may occur. Because symptoms may not be apparent, see your doctor for an examination regularly. |
| Dyrenium or Dyazide/ Potassium Supplements | A | The amount of potassium in your blood may become excessive and thereby lead to disturbances in heart fuction. Keep appointments to have your potassium checked regularly. |
| Lasix/Charcoal | A | Medications for intestinal gas that contain charcoal may reduce the absorption of Lasix into the blood-stream. Lasix may be less effective. Take Lasix two hours before medications that contain charcoal. |
| Lasix/Lithium | D | See Key 24. |
| Lasix/NSAIDs | C | Lasix may be less effective in lowering your blood pressure. Your doctor may adjust your Lasix dosage or change the pain reliever. |
| Midamor or Moduretic/ ACE Inhibitors | D | The amount of potassium in your blood could increase. Your doctor may want you to have your potassium blood level checked regularly. |
| Midamor or Moduretic/ Potassium Supplements | A | The amount of potassium in your blood may become excessive and thereby lead to disturbances in heart function. Keep appointments to have your potassium checked regularly. |
| Thiazides/ Anticoagulants | D | See Key 19. |
| Thiazides/Calcium | B | See Key 41. |
| Thiazides/Diabetes Medicines | C | See Key 28. |
| Thiazides/Lithium | A | See Key 24. |

| Drug Interaction | Rating* | Potential Effects/Recommendations |
|---|---|---|
| Thiazides/Questran | C | The thiazide diurectic may be less effective. Questran binds with thiazide diuretics in the intestinal tract, thereby reducing the absorption of thiazides. Take your diuretic at least 2 hours before Questran. |
| Thiazides/TUMS | B | See Key 36. |
| Thiazides/Zyloprim | B | You may experience side effects such as rash, fever, chills, and intense itching. Contact your doctor *immediately* if you experience this symptoms. |

\* The rating indicates how harmful a drug interaction may be and how frequently it may occur.

"A" indicates a drug interaction that may cause serious harm and occurs frequently. "B" indicates a drug interaction that may cause serious harm but occurs less frequently. "C" indicates a drug interaction that is less harmful but occurs frequently. "D" indicates a drug interaction that is less harmful and occurs less frequently. See Key 9 for more information about the rating system.

# 14

## THE BETA BLOCKERS

The *beta blockers* are used for the treatment of many different medical conditions, such as high blood pressure and rapid heartbeat, as well as for the prevention of heart attack and angina pectoris (chest pain related to clogged arteries of the heart) and of migraine headaches.

### The Medications

There are two major categories of beta blockers:

1. nonselective beta blockers: *Blocadren, Cartrol, Corgard, Inderal, Levatol, Normadyne, propranolol, Trandate,* and *Visken.*
2. cardioselective beta blockers: *Brevibloc, Kerlone, Lopressor, Sectral,* and *Tenormin.*

Both categories of beta blockers act directly on the heart muscle to slow the heart rate, reduce blood pressure, and minimize angina which can lead to heart attack. However, the nonselective beta blockers may also act in other areas of the body, such as the lungs and the arteries.

Inderal, the nonselective beta blocker commonly used to prevent migraine headaches, acts on blood vessels within the brain to reduce the frequency and severity of these headaches.

### Side Effects and Drug Interactions

The most common side effects of beta blockers are dizziness, fatigue, and headache. For most people, these side effects are usually mild and temporary (when treatment is begun). A more serious but less likely side effect is *slow pulse rate* (less than 60 beats per minute). If you experience this side effect, you should contact your doctor as soon as possible.

If you have glanced through the drug interaction charts throughout the book, you may have noticed that drug interactions are more likely to occur with the nonselective than with the cardioselective beta blockers. The reason is that the nonselective beta blockers tend to act not only on the heart muscle but also in the lungs and arteries. Because of their action in the lungs, nonselective beta blockers are more likely to interfere with asthma or chronic obstructive pulmonary disease (COPD) medications thereby worsening such symptoms as wheezing, coughing, and chest congestion.

Inderal and Lopressor may be less effective if combined with medications that increase their metabolism (breakdown into inactive products). Other beta blockers are less likely to be affected by the same medications because these beta blockers follow a different route within the body.

There is one thing you should not do when you are taking a beta blocker: *Do not skip doses or suddenly stop taking the beta blocker* without your doctor's permission. Doing so may worsen your condition and increase the risk of serious heart abnormalities. Remember to refill your beta-blocker prescription before it runs out, and be sure to take sufficient quantities when traveling.

## DRUG INTERACTION CHART:
## THE BETA BLOCKERS

| Drug Interaction | Rating* | Potential Effects/Recommendations |
|---|---|---|
| Beta Blockers/ Antacids | D | Inderal or Tenormin may not be completely absorbed. Take the antacid two hours before or after the beta blocker. |
| Beta Blockers/ Apresoline | B | Both drugs may be more potent. These medications are often combined intentionally to reduce blood pressure. |
| Beta Blockers/ Barbiturates | C | Inderal or Lopressor may be less effective when combined with a barbiturate. Your doctor may adjust your beta blocker dosage. |
| Beta Blockers/Brethine | C | See Key 20. |

| Drug Interaction | Rating* | Potential Effects/Recommendations |
|---|---|---|
| Beta Blockers/ Calcium Tablets | C | Tenormin may be less effective. Your Tenormin dosage may have to be adjusted. |
| Beta Blockers/ Cardizem | D | Inderal or Lopressor may have a more potent effect. Your doctor may adjust the dosage of the beta blocker, or change to Tenormin, a beta blocker that does not interact with Cardizem. |
| Beta Blockers/Catapres | A | See Key 12. |
| Beta Blockers/ Darvon or Darvocet-N | D | Inderal or Lopressor may have a slightly more potent effect. If you feel dizzy, light-headed, and excessively tired, call your doctor. |
| Beta Blockers/ Decongestants | B | Cold/allergy medications that contain phenylephrine may result in increased blood pressure. Ask your doctor whether you can take deconges- tants with your beta blocker. |
| Beta Blockers/Food | C | Inderal and Lopressor are absorbed more completely and may have a slightly more potent effect. This *does not* mean that you have to take Inderal or Lopressor with food. However, you should be consistent; if you like to take your medication with breakfast, try to take it with breakfast every day. |
| Beta Blockers/Insulin | A | See Key 28. |
| Beta Blockers/Isuprel | A | See Key 20. |
| Beta Blockers/Lithium | D | See Key 24. |
| Beta Blockers/ Minipress | A | See Key 12. |
| Beta Blockers/NSAIDs | C | The beta blocker may be less effective, especially if combined with Indocin. Clinoril is less likely to interact. |

| Drug Interaction | Rating* | Potential Effects/Recommendations |
|---|---|---|
| Beta Blockers/ Procardia (Adalat) | D | This combination is often prescribed to treat people who have both high blood pressure and angina. However, slow pulse rate and very low blood pressure can occur in some people. If you feel dizzy, light-headed, and excessively tired, call your doctor. |
| Beta Blockers/Quinidine | D | In some people, Inderal or Lopressor may have a more potent action. Inderal and quinidine are often used together. Your doctor may examine you frequently when you first start this combined drug treatment. |
| Beta Blockers/Rifampin | A | Inderal or Lopressor may be less effective. Your doctor may adjust your dosage of the beta blocker. |
| Beta Blockers/Tagamet | A | You may experience side effects caused by Inderal or Lopressor (slow pulse rate—less than 60 beats per minute). Your doctor may adjust the dosage of the beta blocker or may replace Tagamet with another ulcer drug. |
| Beta Blockers/ Theophylline | A | See Key 20. |
| Inderal/Colestid | B | Inderal may be less effective. Take Inderal 2 hours before or after Colestid. Your doctor may have to adjust your Inderal dosage. |
| Inderal/Digoxin | B | People who unknowingly have high blood levels of digoxin may be at higher risk for developing slow heart rate. Your doctor may want to check your digoxin blood level periodically. If you feel dizzy, light-headed, and excessively tired, call your doctor. |
| Inderal/Haldol | B | Both drugs may have more potent effect. Your doctor may adjust the dosages of both medications. |

| Drug Interaction | Rating* | Potential Effects/Recommendations |
|---|---|---|
| Inderal/Migraine Headache Medications That Contain Ergotamine (Cafergot, Ergomar, Sansert) | B | This combination is often used to treat migraine headache attacks. Side effects can occur but are rare. If your hands or feet feel extremely cold, become numb, or turn purple or blue, contact your doctor *immediately*. |
| Inderal/Neo-Synephrine Nasal Spray | B | Excessive doses of Neo-Synephrine may lead to a sudden increase in blood pressure. Ask your doctor whether you may use Neo-Synephrine while taking Inderal. |
| Inderal/Questran | D | Inderal may be less effective. Take Inderal two hours before or after Questran. Your doctor may have to adjust your Inderal dosage. |
| Inderal/Thorazine | A | Both drugs may have more potent effects. Your doctor may adjust the dosage of both medications. |
| Lopressor/Calan | A | Lopressor may have a more potent action which could lead to side effects that involve the heart. Your doctor will probably want to examine you frequently when you start this combination. |

\* The rating indicates how harmful a drug interaction may be and how frequently it may occur.

"A" indicates a drug interaction that may cause serious harm and occurs frequently. "B" indicates a drug interaction that may cause serious harm but occurs less frequently. "C" indicates a drug interaction that is less harmful but occurs frequently. "D" indicates a drug interaction that is less harmful and occurs less frequently. See Key 9 for more information about the rating system.

# 15

## HEART MEDICATIONS
## FOR ANGINA

*Angina pectoris* is a condition in which blood flow through the heart is drastically reduced, resulting in chest pain that may radiate through the left arm. Reduced blood flow may be caused by blockages in the coronary arteries, or may occur if the openings through the coronary arteries are too narrow for the blood to flow through. A heart attack may occur if blood flow through these arteries stops completely.

### The Medications

Three categories of medications are used to prevent and/or relieve symptoms of angina:

1. nitrates: *Cardilate, Isordil, Peritrate,* and all forms of *nitroglycerin,* such as *Nitro-Bid* capsules, *Nitrostat* sublingual tablets, *Nitro-Dur* or *Transderm-Nitro* patches, and *Nitro-Bid* or *Nitrol* ointment.
2. calcium channel blockers: *Adalat, Calan, Cardene, Cardizem, Dynacirc, Isoptin, nifedipine, Nimotop, Procardia, Vascor, verapamil,* and *Verelan.*
3. beta blockers, discussed in Key 14.

### Side Effects and Drug Interactions

**Nitrates**
If you have ever taken a nitroglycerin tablet under your tongue, you may have experienced a slight headache and a stinging sensation in your mouth where the tablet dissolved. In fact, your doctor may have told you, "When you feel those symptoms, you know the drug is working!"

The most frequent side effect of the nitrates is headache, which can be severe. Other side effects are dizziness, weakness, increased heart rate, and nausea. Combining the nitrate with an alcoholic beverage may intensify these side effects. Therefore, you should ask your doctor if you may drink alcoholic beverages while taking a nitrate.

Hydergine and ergotamine (a drug in migraine headache products) are two medications that may interfere with the action of nitrates because their action is *opposite* to that of the nitrates. Therefore, these drugs may cause increased anginal symptoms.

### Calcium Channel Blocker

The most common side effects of the calcium channel blockers (CCBs) are dizziness, light-headedness, headache, nausea, constipation, and edema. These side effects may become more pronounced if you take another medication that increases the potency of the CCB. The drug interaction between Procardia and Tagamet is a good example.

Some medications may reduce the effectiveness of nitrates or calcium channel blockers. With such combinations, increased symptoms of angina may occur.

### Beta Blockers

For side effects and drug interactions of beta blockers, see Key 14.

## DRUG INTERACTION CHART: HEART MEDICATIONS FOR ANGINA

All of the calcium channel blockers (CCBs) interact with certain other medications similarly, so they are listed as a group. The same is true of the nitrates. Drug interactions that involve specific CCBs are discussed separately.

| Drug Interaction | Rating* | Potential Effects/Recommendations |
| --- | --- | --- |
| Calan/Digoxin | A | See Key 17. |
| Calan SR/Food | C | Sustained action Calan (Isoptin) should be taken with meals to ensure consistent blood levels of the drug. |
| Calan/Quinidine | A | See Key 16. |

| Drug Interaction | Rating* | Potential Effects/Recommendations |
|---|---|---|
| Calan/Theophylline | B | See Key 20. |
| CCBs/Alcohol | A | If you are taking Calan, you may become intoxicated more quickly and to a greater extent. Intoxication may last for a prolonged period of time. |
| CCBs/Calcium Supplements (Oscal, Citracal) | C | All of the CCBs may become less effective. Before taking a calcium supplement, ask your doctor whether it will interfere with your CCB treatment. |
| CCBs/Lithium | A | See Key 24. |
| CCBs/Minipress | A | See Key 12. |
| CCBs/Phenobarbital | A | Calan or Procardia may be less effective. Your doctor may adjust the dosage of Calan or Procardia when you start phenobarbital. |
| CCBs/Sandimmune | A | See Key 34. |
| CCBs/Tegretol | A | See Key 30. |
| CCBs/TUMS | C | The CCBs may be less effective. Ask your pharmacist to help you select an antacid that does not contain calcium. |
| Cardizem/Digoxin | D | See Key 17. |
| Cardizem/Tagamet | D | You may experience Cardizem side effects (headache, nausea, dizziness). Your doctor may adjust your Cardizem dosage. |
| Cardizem/Theophylline | D | See Key 20. |
| Cardizem/Zantac | D | Cardizem may have a more potent effect. Contact your doctor if you experience headache, dizziness, or nausea. The dosage of Cardizem may have to be adjusted. |
| Nitrates/Alcohol | A | Alcohol may intensify the effects of nitrates. You may feel dizzy, weak, or faint. |
| Nitrates/Hydergine | A | Your angina may worsen. If it does, tell your doctor *immediately*. |

| Drug Interaction | Rating* | Potential Effects/Recommendations |
|---|---|---|
| Nitrates/Migraine Headache Medications That Contain Ergotamine | A | Your angina may worsen. Do not take this combination without first checking with your doctor. |
| Nitroglycerin Sublingual/Aspirin | D | You may develop a headache, weakness, and dizziness. Ask your doctor what dosage of aspirin you can take. |
| Procardia/Quinidine | D | Procardia may be less effective. Your doctor may replace Procardia with another medication that does not interact with quinidine, such as Cardizem. |
| Procardia/Tagamet | A | Procardia may have a more potent effect. If you experience palpitations or a pulse rate over 100 beats per minute, contact your doctor. |
| Procardia/ Theophylline | D | See Key 20. |

* The rating indicates how harmful a drug interaction may be and how frequently it may occur.

"A" indicates a drug interaction that may cause serious harm and occurs frequently. "B" indicates a drug interaction that may cause serious harm but occurs less frequently. "C" indicates a drug interaction that is less harmful but occurs frequently. "D" indicates a drug interaction that is less harmful and occurs less frequently. See Key 9 for more information about the rating system.

# 16

## HEART MEDICATIONS
## FOR ARRHYTHMIAS

The heart muscle is made up of four chambers, all which contract in a special order and rhythm. *Arrhythmias* (irregular or abnormal heartbeat) may occur when one or more of these chambers contract "out of sync" from the other chambers. When this happens, the heart muscle cannot contract properly to pump blood to the rest of the body.

There are many different types of arrhythmias, depending on which chamber or chambers are contracting out of sync. Symptoms vary depending on the type of arrhythmia. If you are being treated for an arrhythmia, ask your doctor what symptoms you should be aware of. You can then let your doctor know if your arrhythmia condition is getting worse, or if your symptoms intensify when another medication is added to your treatment.

### The Medications

The most common medications used to treat arrhythmias are *Bretylol, Cordarone, Decabid, disopyramide, Enkaid, Ethmozine, Mexitil, Norpace, Procan, procainamide, Pronestyl, Quinidine, Rythmol, Tambocor,* and *Tonocard.* Other medications prescribed to treat arrhythmias are the beta blockers (Key 14) and *digoxin* (Key 17).

### Side Effects and Drug Interactions

Arrhythmias are sometimes difficult to treat because the medications that are available tend to cause side effects, some of which can be serious. *Medication dosing is critical.* If the amount of medication in the bloodstream gets too high (the drug is too potent), side effects are more likely to occur. If the

45

amount of medication in the bloodstream is too low, the drug may be less effective or even ineffective, and the arrhythmia symptoms may worsen.

To ensure that you are getting the correct dosage, your doctor may want to check your medication blood level (the amount of drug in the blood) regularly. If your medication dosage is too high, or if you start taking an additional drug that causes your arrhythmia medication to have a more potent action, your blood level may increase, thereby increasing the likelihood of side effects.

Listed below are some arrhythmia medications and their most common side effects. With increased drug potency, these signs and symptoms may be more pronounced.

1. *Cordarone:* fatigue, nausea, reduced coordination, and visual symptoms.
2. *Ethmozine:* dizziness, headache, fatigue, nausea, shortness of breath, and palpitations.
3. *Procainamide (Procan):* nausea, vomiting, diarrhea and itching.
4. *Quinidine:* ringing in the ears, headache, nausea, dizziness, and in severe cases, abnormal heartbeat.
5. *Tambocor:* dizziness, visual disturbances, headache, nausea, fatigue, shortness of breath, and palpitations.

The one arrhythmia medication that is affected by food is Rythmol. The presence of food in the intestine may increase the amount of Rythmol absorbed into the bloodstream and thereby lead to unwanted side effects. Therefore, it is important to be consistent in the way you take Rythmol each day. If you like to take the medication with meals, always do so; if you like to take it on an empty stomach, do so for each dose. If you are consistent in the way you take the drug, your doctor can more easily adjust the dosage if you experience side effects or lack of Rythmol effectiveness.

Keep in mind that proper dosing is critical for these medications. Therefore, it is especially important that you do not skip doses.

## DRUG INTERACTION CHART:
## HEART MEDICATIONS FOR ARRYTHMIAS

| Drug Interaction | Rating* | Potential Effects/Recommendations |
|---|---|---|
| Enkaid/Quinidine | B | In a few people, Enkaid may have a more potent effect. Your Enkaid blood level may be checked frequently when you start taking both medications together. |
| Mexitil/Dilantin | A | Mexitil may be less effective if taken with Dilantin. Your doctor may adjust your dosage of Mexitil. |
| Mexitil/Rifampin | A | Mexitil may lose effectiveness and your heart condition may worsen. Your doctor may adjust your Mexitil dosage when rifampin is started or discontinued. |
| Mexitil/Theophylline | A | See Key 20. |
| Norpace/Dilantin | C | See Key 30. |
| Norpace/Erythromycin | B | Although rare, Norpace side effects are possible when erythromycin is combined with Norpace. |
| Norpace/Phenobarbital | A | Norpace may be less effective. Your doctor may want to check your Norpace blood level when you start or discontinue phenobarital. Be sure to keep your appointment for lab work. |
| Norpace/Rifampin | A | Norpace may be less effective. Your doctor may want to check your Norpace blood level when you start or discontinue rifampin. Be sure to keep your appointment for lab work. |
| Procan/Bactrim or Septra | B | You may experience Procan side effects (nausea, vomiting, diarrhea, itching). Contact your doctor if you experience these symptoms. |
| Procan/Quinidine | D | Procan may have a more potent effect. Your doctor may want to check your Procan blood level regularly. |

47

| Drug Interaction | Rating* | Potential Effects/Recommendations |
|---|---|---|
| Procan/Tagamet | A | Procan may have a more potent effect, and you may experience Procan side effects. Your doctor may adjust your Procan dosage. |
| Procan/Zantac | B | Procan may have a more potent effect, and you may experience Procan side effects. Your doctor may adjust your Procan dosage. |
| Quinidine/Antacids | A | Quinidine may have a more potent effect when combined with some antacids. Amphogel and Alternagel are two antacids that are less likely to interact with quinidine. |
| Quinidine/Barbiturates | A | Quinidine may lose effectiveness. Your doctor may adjust your quinidine dosage. |
| Quinidine/Beta Blockers | D | See Key 14. |
| Quinidine/Calan (Isoptin) | A | You may experience side effects that involve the heart and circulatory blood system. It is important that you keep your appointments to have your quinidine blood level checked regularly. |
| Quinidine/Coumadin | B | See Key 19. |
| Quinidine/Diamox | B | Quinidine may have a more potent effect. Your doctor may want to check your quinidine blood level when you start or discontinue Diamox. |
| Quinidine/Digoxin | A | See Key 17. |
| Quinidine/Dilantin | A | Quinidine may be less effective. Your doctor may want to check your quinidine blood level if your Dilantin dosage changes. Be sure to keep your appointment for lab work. |

| Drug Interaction | Rating* | Potential Effects/Recommendations |
|---|---|---|
| Quinidine/Kaopectate | C | Quinidine may not be completely absorbed into the bloodstream and may therefore be less effective. To minimize this interaction, take these medications several hours apart. |
| Quinidine/Mysoline | A | Quinidine may be less effective. Your doctor may adjust the quinidine dosage. |
| Quinidine/Nizoral | B | Quinidine may have a more potent effect. Your doctor may want to check your quinidine blood level when your start or discontinue Nizoral treatment. |
| Quinidine/Procardia | D | See Key 15. |
| Quinidine/Rifampin | A | Quinidine may have a more potent effect. Your doctor may want to check your quinidine blood level when you start or discontinue rifampin. |
| Quinidine/Tagamet | A | You may experience quinidine side effects, especially when you start quinidine treatment. Your doctor may want to check your quinidine blood level regularly. Be sure to keep your appointment for lab work. |
| Quinidine/TCAs | A | See Key 23. |

\* The rating indicates how harmful a drug interaction may be and how frequently it may occur.

"A" indicates a drug interaction that may cause serious harm and occurs frequently. "B" indicates a drug interaction that may cause serious harm but occurs less frequently. "C" indicates a drug interaction that is less harmful but occurs frequently. "D" indicates a drug interaction that is less harmful and occurs less frequently. See Key 9 for more information about the rating system.

# 17

# DIGOXIN—INVOLVED IN MANY DRUG INTERACTIONS

*Digoxin* is a medication used to treat different kinds of heart abnormalities. However, it is most often prescribed for *congestive heart failure*, a condition in which the heart muscle does not contract with enough force to pump blood to the rest of the body.

## The Medications

*Digoxin* is a member of the *digitalis* class of drugs. You may be more familiar with digoxin's brand name, *Lanoxin*. Digoxin is also available in capsules called *Lanoxicaps*.

## Side Effects and Drug Interactions

Digoxin is a potent medication; only a very small amount of the drug (0.125 or 0.25 mg) is needed to produce its action. Compare this to one aspirin tablet, which contains 325 mg of aspirin!

Most important, there is precious little margin for error with digoxin—a little too much or not quite enough drug in the bloodstream can cause too potent an effect or not enough effect, respectively. Therefore, any change in the way digoxin is absorbed into the bloodstream or in the way it is handled in the body can alter its effectiveness.

If digoxin is combined with another medication that *increases the potency* of digoxin, you may experience side effects such as nausea, vomiting, anorexia, diarrhea, headache, weakness, heart abnormalities, and visual effects (green or yellow halos around objects and blurred vision). If digoxin is combined with another medication that causes digoxin to be *less effective*, your heart condition may worsen, a situation that may produce symptoms. Either way, you should contact your doctor *immediately* if you experience any symptoms that may be related to the drug or your heart condition.

To reduce the chance of digoxin side effects or lack of effectiveness, your doctor may want to check the amount of digoxin in your bloodstream. This is done by taking a sample of blood and measuring the concentration of digoxin in the blood to get a final number referred to as the *blood level*. If the blood level is within a certain range, your digoxin dosage is right for you. If your digoxin blood level is too high or too low (out of the specified range), your doctor may adjust your digoxin dosage.

In the digoxin drug interaction chart in this Key, I sometimes recommend that you ask your pharmacist to give you the brand-name product, Lanoxin, instead of the generic substitute. My reason is that Lanoxin, unlike some of the other generic brands, does not interact with certain other medications.

Why do some brands of digoxin interact with a particular drug, such as Reglan, and other brands do not? The answer is that Lanoxin dissolves, disintegrates, and is absorbed into the bloodstream before Reglan pushes it into the large intestine, where it is not well absorbed. Other brands of digoxin may not be absorbed in time and may lose their effectiveness. Therefore, for these kinds of drug combinations, I recommend the brand name over the generic substitute. (This is not true, however, for other generic medications, which have been shown to be just as effective as their brand-name counterparts, and can save you money.)

# DRUG INTERACTION CHART:
## DIGOXIN—INVOLVED IN MANY
## DRUG INTERACTIONS

| Drug Interaction | Rating* | Potential Effects/Recommendations |
|---|---|---|
| Digoxin/ACE Inhibitors | D | Digoxin may have a more potent effect. Your doctor may want to check your digoxin blood level regularly. Be sure to keep your appointments for lab work. |
| Digoxin/Aldactone | B | Digoxin may have a more potent action. It is important that you keep your appointments with your doctor so that you can be examined for digoxin side effects—in this case, lab work may not be enough. |
| Digoxin/Antispasmodics | B | Digoxin tablets may have a more potent action. Lanoxin (the brand-name product) is not affected, so ask your pharmacist to fill your prescription with Lanoxin instead of the generic substitute. |
| Digoxin/Antacids | C | Antacids may reduce the absorption of digoxin into the bloodstream; digoxin may be less effective. Take digoxin two hours before or after the antacid. |
| Digoxin/Azulfidine | B | Azulfidine may be less effective. Take digoxin two hours before or after Azulfidine. |
| Digoxin/Calan | A | You may experience side effects of digoxin. Contact your doctor *as soon as possible* if you do. Your doctor may want to check your digoxin blood level regularly. Be sure to keep your appointments for lab work. |
| Digoxin/Carafate | D | Digoxin may not be completely absorbed and therefore may be less effective. Take digoxin two hours before or after Carafate. |

| Drug Interaction | Rating* | Potential Effects/Recommendations |
|---|---|---|
| Digoxin/Cardizem | D | Digoxin may have a slightly more potent effect. Your doctor may want to check your digoxin blood level periodically. Be sure to keep your appointment for lab work. |
| Digoxin/Charcoal Capsules | A | Digoxin may be ineffective; charcoal may prevent the absorption of digoxin into the bloodstream. Ask your pharmacist to help you choose another product to relieve intestinal gas. |
| Digoxin/Citrate of Magnesia | D | Digoxin may be less effective if you take excessive amounts of Citrate of Magnesia. Ask your pharmacist to help you select another laxative that does not contain magnesium. |
| Digoxin/Colestid | A | Digoxin may lose its effectivness because it binds with Colestid in the gastrointestinal tract and does not become absorbed into the bloodstream. Take digoxin two hours before or after Colestid. |
| Digoxin/Diabetes Medicines | D | Digoxin may have a slightly more potent effect if combined with Ornase, Diabeta, or Micronase. Your doctor may want to check your digoxin blood levels periodically. Be sure to keep your appointments for lab work. |
| Digoxin/Dilantin | D | Digoxin may be less effective. Your doctor may want to check your blood level regularly. |
| Digoxin/Diuretics | B | Diuretics that reduce the amount of potassium in the bloodstream, such as Lasix, Bumex, Edecrin, and the thiazides, may increase the risk of digoxin side effects. It is important that you keep your appointments to have your digoxin blood level checked regularly. |

| Drug Interaction | Rating* | Potential Effects/Recommendations |
|---|---|---|
| Digoxin/Erythromycin | B | Digoxin may have a more potent effect (approximately 10 percent of people). Contact your doctor if you experience digoxin side effects. |
| Digoxin/Ibuprofen | D | Digoxin may have a more potent effect if you take large doses of ibuprofen every day. Your doctor may want to check your digoxin blood level regularly. |
| Digoxin/Inderal | B | See Key 14. |
| Digoxin/Kaopectate | C | Digoxin tablets may not be absorbed as well and may be less effective. Take Kaopectate two hours before or after digoxin. (Digoxin capsules are not affected.) |
| Digoxin/Methotrexate | B | Digoxin tablets may be less effective because they are not completely absorbed. (Digoxin capsules, *Lanoxicaps*, are not affected.) |
| Digoxin/Midamor or Moduretic | B | Digoxin may be less effective. Be sure to keep your appointments with your doctor so that you can be examined regularly. Digoxin blood levels may not be enough. |
| Digoxin/Milk of Magnesia | D | Digoxin may be less effective if you take excessive amounts of Milk of Magnesia. Ask your pharmacist to help you select another laxative that does not contain magnesium. |
| Digoxin/Minocin | B | Digoxin may have a more potent effect (approximately 10% of people). Contact your doctor if you experience digoxin side effects. |
| Digoxin/Propylthiouricil (PTU) | A | The effectiveness of digoxin may change depending on your thyroid condition. |

| Drug Interaction | Rating* | Potential Effects/Recommendations |
|---|---|---|
| Digoxin/Proventil (Ventolin) | B | Digoxin may be less effective. Your doctor may want to check your digoxin blood level periodically. Be sure to keep your appointments for lab work. |
| Digoxin/Questran | A | Digoxin may be less effective; it binds with Questran in the gastrointestinal tract and is not completely absorbed. Take digoxin two hours before or after Questran. |
| Digoxin/Quinidine | A | You may experience side effects of digoxin. If you do, contact your doctor *immediately*. Your doctor may want to check your digoxin blood level regularly. Be sure to keep your appointments for lab work. |
| Digoxin/Quinine (in Q-Vel, Legatrin) | B | You may experience side effects of digoxin. Check with your doctor before combining these medications. |
| Digoxin/Reglan | B | Some brands of digoxin may become less effective. Ask your pharmacist for the brand-name product, Lanoxin, instead of generic digoxin. |
| Digoxin/Rifampin | B | Digoxin may be less effective. Your doctor may adjust the digoxin dosage while you are taking rifampin. |
| Digoxin/Sandimmune | A | You may experience side effects of digoxin. Your doctor may want to check your digoxin blood level regularly. Be sure to keep your appointments for lab work. |
| Digoxin/Tagamet | D | Digoxin may be more potent or less effective when you start or stop Tagamet. Your doctor may adjust your digoxin dosage. |
| Digoxin/Tapazole | A | The effectiveness of digoxin may change, depending on your thyroid condition. |

55

| Drug Interaction | Rating* | Potential Effects/Recommendations |
| --- | --- | --- |
| Digoxin/Tetracycline | B | Digoxin may have a more potent effect (approximately 10 percent of people). Contact your doctor if you experience digoxin side effects. |
| Digoxin/Thyroid Hormone | A | The effectiveness of digoxin may change, depending on your thyroid condition. |
| Digoxin/Valium or Digoxin/Xanax | B | You may experience digoxin side effects when digoxin is combined with Valium or Xanax. If you do, contact your doctor. Your digoxin dosage may have to be adjusted. |
| Digoxin/Vibramycin | B | Digoxin may have a more potent effect (approximately 10 percent of people). Contact your doctor if you experience digoxin side effects. |

* The rating indicates how harmful a drug interaction may be and how frequently it may occur.

"A" indicates a drug interaction that may cause serious harm and occurs frequently. "B" indicates a drug interaction that may cause serious harm but occurs less frequently. "C" indicates a drug interaction that is less harmful but occurs frequently. "D" indicates a drug interaction that is less harmful and occurs less frequently. See Key 9 for more information about the rating system.

# 18

# MEDICATIONS THAT REDUCE CHOLESTEROL

*Cholesterol* is a form of fat that carries out many functions in the body. Cholesterol not only is manufactured by the body, but also is found in many foods. The recently publicized connection between cholesterol and heart disease has sent many people running for cholesterol screening tests to find out whether their cholesterol blood levels put them at higher risk for heart ailments.

## The Medications

Medications used to treat high cholesterol are *Atromid S, Cholixin, Cholybar, Colestid, Lopid, Lorelco, Mevacor,* and *Questran.*

Treatment for reducing cholesterol may involve just a low cholesterol diet. Some people, however, cannot reduce their cholesterol levels with diet alone and may also have to take medication. Drug treatment usually involves one medication, but in some cases a combination of cholesterol medications may be needed.

## Side Effects and Drug Interactions

Questran and Colestid are usually not affected by other medications. However, they do interfere with the actions of other medications by binding to them, thereby preventing their absorption into the bloodstream, with a possible loss of their effectiveness. To prevent this kind of drug interaction, take your other medication one or two hours before Questran or Colestid.

Atromid S and Mevacor are affected by other medications, which can cause increased potency in each of these drugs.

57

Muscle weakness or muscle pain may be an indication that your Atromid S or Mevacor dosage is too high. If you experience these symptoms, call your doctor because your dosage may have to be adjusted.

Your doctor may want to check the effectiveness of your treatment by checking your cholesterol level periodically. Since this is an important step in determining whether the medication and the dosage you are taking are right for you, be sure to keep your appointments for cholesterol-level checkups.

There are three things you should remember when you take your cholesterol medication:

1. If you are taking Questran or Cholybar, be sure to drink plenty of water; this will help minimize constipation. Always take Questran powder mixed with a glassful of juice or a bowlful of soup or cereal, not by itself. Take Questran or Cholybar with meals to reduce upset stomach and to increase the drug's effectiveness.

2. If you are taking Mevacor, take it with your evening meal to enhance its absorption (unless your doctor tells you otherwise).

3. It is important that you stick faithfully to your low-cholesterol diet—cholesterol medications are not a substitute for proper diet.

## DRUG INTERACTION CHART:
## MEDICATIONS THAT REDUCE CHOLESTEROL

| Drug Interaction | Rating* | Potential Effects/Recommendations |
|---|---|---|
| Atromid S/ Anticoagulants | A | See Key 19. |
| Atromid S/Benemid | D | Atromid S may have a more potent effect. Contact your doctor if you experience Atromid side effects such as muscle pain or weakness. |
| Atromid S/Diabetes Medicines | D | See Key 28. |

| Drug Interaction | Rating* | Potential Effects/Recommendations |
|---|---|---|
| Atromid S/Estrogens | D | Atromid S may be less effective. Your doctor may want you to have your cholesterol level checked periodically. |
| Cholixin/Coumadin | A | See Key 19. |
| Colestid/Digoxin | A | See Key 17. |
| Colestid/Inderal | B | See Key 14. |
| Colestid/ The Tetracyclines | B | See Key 31. |
| Lopid/Colestid | D | Lopid may be less effective if taken at the same time as Colestid. Take Lopid two hours before or after Colestid. |
| Mevacor/Erythromycin | B | Mevacor may have a more potent effect. Contact your doctor *immediately* if you experience side effects of Mevacor, such as muscle pain or weakness. |
| Mevacor/Food | C | Mevacor is best absorbed when taken with the evening meal. |
| Mevacor/Lopid | A | You may experience side effects caused by Mevacor such as muscle pain or weakness. If you do, contact your doctor *immediately*. |
| Mevacor/Niacin | B | You may experience side effects of Mevacor, such as muscle pain or weakness. Before you start taking nonprescription niacin, ask your doctor to recommend a dosage that will not interfere with your Mevacor treatment. |
| Mevacor/Sandimmune | A | You may experience side effects caused by Mevacor such as muscle pain or weakness. If you do, contact your doctor immediately. |
| Mevacor/Thyroid Hormone | B | See Key 29. |
| Questran/ Acetaminophen | C | See Key 35. |

| Drug Interaction | Rating* | Potential Effects/Recommendations |
|---|---|---|
| Questran/Coumadin | A | See Key 19. |
| Questran/Digoxin | A | See Key 17. |
| Questran/Flagyl | D | See Key 31. |
| Questran/Food | A | Take Questran with meals to enhance its effectiveness. |
| Questran/Hydrocortisone | B | See Key 29. |
| Questran/Inderal | D | See Key 14. |
| Questran/Methotrexate | A | See Key 33. |
| Questran/Thiazides | C | See Key 13. |
| Questran/Thyroid Hormone | A | See Key 29. |

\* The rating indicates how harmful a drug interaction may be and how frequently it may occur.

"A" indicates a drug interaction that may cause serious harm and occurs frequently. "B" indicates a drug interaction that may cause serious harm but occurs less frequently. "C" indicates a drug interaction that is less harmful but occurs frequently. "D" indicates a drug interaction that is less harmful and occurs less frequently. See Key 9 for more information about the rating system.

# 19

## ANTICOAGULANTS (BLOOD THINNERS)

*Anticoagulants*, commonly known as "blood thinners," are medications that prevent the blood from clotting or delay clotting. They are prescribed most often to prevent the formation (or worsening) of blood clots in the arteries of the heart or lungs.

### The Medications

Anticoagulant drug treatment usually begins while the heart-attack victim is in the hospital, with *heparin*, an injectable anticoagulant. After the right dosage of heparin (which is individualized for each person), has been determined, the person is usually ready to be switched from heparin to *Coumadin* tablets. (The generic name for Coumadin is *warfarin*.) Another commonly prescribed anticoagulant is *dicumarol*.

### Side Effects and Drug Interactions

The most important "side effect" that can occur if you skip doses of your anticoagulant is a lack of effectiveness, which can lead to increased danger of blood clots. Conversely, one possible side effect if you take too much or inadvertently take extra doses of the anticoagulant is hemorrhage (excessive bleeding), which is also dangerous. You can see how important it is to follow your dosage schedule exactly as your doctor has prescribed.

Increases in potency (and danger of bleeding) or decreases in effectiveness (and danger of blood clots) can also occur when other medications interfere with the action of anticoagulants.

Of all the drugs in the pharmacy, Coumadin and dicumarol are probably the two that interact most with other medications, mainly because these anticoagulants bind extensively to proteins that circulate in the blood. These blood proteins actually act as "drug reservoirs." (See Key 6 for an explanation of how "protein binding" may affect a medication's action.)

When an oral anticoagulant is attached to its blood protein "reservoir," it is not available to produce *any* effect. For this reason enough drug must be available in the bloodstream both to bind with proteins in the blood *and* to fight blood clots. With the proper doasage, just enough Coumadin is "freed" from its binding protein to produce its clot-fighting action. However, an interacting drug may dislodge too much Coumadin from the protein, thereby freeing it to produce too potent an effect.

To make sure that your anticoagulant dosage is right for you, your doctor may want to do a blood test that measures the amount of time required for your blood to clot. This blood test, referred to as a "prothrombin time" (PT), will alert your doctor if the dosage is too high or low. On the basis of the results of the test, your doctor may adjust your anticoagulant dosage.

### DRUG INTERACTION CHART: ANTICOAGULANTS (BLOOD THINNERS)

| Drug Interaction | Rating* | Potential Effects/Recommendations |
| --- | --- | --- |
| Anticoagulants/ Alcohol | D | The anticoagulant may have a more potent effect if you drink enough alcohol to become intoxicated. Ask your doctor whether you can drink alcoholic beverages while being treated with the anticoagulant and if so, what quantity is safe. |
| Anticoagulants/Aspirin | A | The anticoagulant may have a more potent effect. Even a small dosage of aspirin can lead to anticoagulant side effects. Check with your doctor before taking any nonprescription medication. If your doctor allows you to take allergy/ cold products, ask your pharmacist to help you select a product that does not contain aspirin. |

| Drug Interaction | Rating* | Potential Effects/Recommendations |
|---|---|---|
| Anticoagulants/ Atromid S | A | The anticoagulant may have a more potent effect. Your doctor may want to check your PT frequently. Be sure not to skip doses of either medication. |
| Anticoagulants/ Barbiturates | A | The anticoagulants may be less effective. If you are taking a barbiturate consistently, (such as phenobarbital for epilepsy), your doctor may adjust the dosage of the anticoagulant. Be sure not to skip doses of either medication. |
| Anticoagulants/ Butazolidin | A | The anticoagulant may have a more potent effect which can lead to side effects. Your doctor may want to check your PT frequently. |
| Anticoagulants/ Corticosteroids | D | The effectiveness of the anticoagulant may be changed if you are taking Decadron or prednisone. Your doctor may adjust your dosage. |
| Anticoagulants/ Cytadren | D | The anticoagulant may be less effective. Your doctor may adjust your dosage when you start or stop Cytadren. |
| Anticoagulants/Dilantin | B | The effectiveness of the anticoagulant may change. Your doctor may want to check your PT regularly. In addition, Dilantin may have a more potent effect when combined with dicumarol. |
| Anticoagulants/Flagyl | A | The anticoagulant may have a more potent effect. Your doctor may want to check your PT while you are taking Flagyl. |
| Anticoagulants/Food | C | The anticoagulant may be less effective if you eat excessive amounts of foods that contain vitamin K, such as asparagus, spinach, broccoli, lettuce, and tomato. Once your anticoagulant dosage has been adjusted, be consistent in the amounts of green leafy vegetables that you eat. (Note: "vitamin |

| Drug Interaction | Rating* | Potential Effects/Recommendations |
|---|---|---|
| | | K" should not be confused with "K," the chemical symbol used for potassium supplement products.) |
| Anticoagulants/ Ibuprofen | D | The anticoagulant may have a more potent effect. Ask your doctor whether you may take ibuprofen and, if so, what dosage is correct. |
| Anticoagulants/ Isoniazid (INH) | D | The anticoagulant may have a more potent effect. Your doctor may check your PT regularly. |
| Anticoagulants/ Minocin | D | The anticoagulant may have a more potent effect, especially in persons who are malnourished. Your doctor may want to check your PT while you are taking Minocin. |
| Anticoagulants/ Mysoline | A | The anticoagulant may be less effective. Your doctor may adjust your dosage. Do not skip doses of either medication because doing so may change the effectiveness of the anticoagulant. |
| Anticoagulants/ NegGram | D | The anticoagulant may have a more potent effect. Your doctor may check your PT while you are taking NegGram. |
| Anticoagulants/NSAIDs | C | The anticoagulant may have a more potent effect. Your doctor may want to check your PT reguarly. |
| Anticoagulants/ Rifampin | A | The anticoagulant may be less effective. Your doctor may adjust your anticoagulant dosage. |
| Anticoagulants/ Propylthiouricil (PTU) | A | The effectiveness of the anticoagulant may change when you start, stop, or change the dosage of PTU. Your doctor may want to check your PT frequently. |
| Anticoagulants/ Tapazole | A | The effectiveness of the anticoagulant may change when you start, stop, or change the dosage of Tapazole. Your doctor may want to check your PT frequently. |

| Drug Interaction | Rating* | Potential Effects/Recommendations |
|---|---|---|
| Anticoagulants/ Tegretol | D | The anticoagulant may be less effective. This interaction may occur a few weeks after you have begun to take both drugs together. Therefore, your doctor may want to check your PT regularly. |
| Anticoagulants/ Tetracycline | D | The anticoagulant may have a more potent effect, especially in persons who are malnourished. Your doctor may want to check your PT while you are taking tetracycline. |
| Anticoagulants/ Thiazide Diuretics | D | The anticoagulant may be less effective. Your doctor may want to check your PT periodically. |
| Anticoagulants/ Thyroid Hormone | A | The effectiveness of the anticoagulant may change when you start, stop, or change the dosage of thyroid hormone. Your doctor may want to check your PT frequently. |
| Anticoagulants/ Vibramycin | D | The anticoagulant may have a more potent effect, especially in persons who are malnourished. Your doctor may want to check your PT while you are taking Vibramycin. |
| Anticoagulants/ Vitamin E | A | The anticoagulant may have a more potent effect. Check with your doctor before you take any vitamin product. |
| Anticoagulants/ Zyloprim | D | Some anticoagulants may have a slightly more potent effect. Coumadin is less likely to interact with Zyloprim. |
| Coumadin/Anturane | A | Coumadin may have a more potent effect. Your doctor may want to check your PT regularly. |
| Coumadin/Carafate | D | Coumadin may be less effective. Take Coumadin at least 2 hours before or after Carafate. |

| Drug Interaction | Rating* | Potential Effects/Recommendations |
|---|---|---|
| Coumadin/Cholixin | A | Coumadin may have a more potent effect. Your doctor may want to check your PT frequently and may adjust your Coumadin dosage. |
| Coumadin/Cipro | D | Coumadin may have a more potent effect. Your doctor may want to check your PT while you are taking Cipro. |
| Coumadin/Cytoxan | D | Coumadin may be less effective. Your doctor may want to check your PT when you start or discontinue Cytoxan. |
| Coumadin/Darvon or Darvocet-N | D | Coumadin may have a slightly more potent effect. Your doctor may want to check your PT regularly. |
| Coumadin/Diflucan | D | Coumadin may have a more potent effect. Your doctor may want to check your PT while you are taking Diflucan. |
| Coumadin/ Erythromycin | C | Coumadin may have a more potent effect. Your doctor may want to check your PT while you are taking erythromycin. |
| Coumadin/Floxin | D | Coumadin may have a more potent effect. Your doctor may want to check your PT while you are taking Floxin. |
| Coumadin/Fulvicin | D | Coumadin may be less effective. Your doctor may adjust your Coumadin dosage. |
| Coumadin/Glucagon | B | Coumadin may have a more potent effect. If you are taking glucagon for more than two days, your doctor may adjust your dosage of Coumadin. |
| Coumadin/Nizoral | B | Coumadin may have a more potent effect. Your doctor may want to check your PT while you are taking Nizoral. |
| Coumadin/Nolvadex | B | Coumadin may have a more potent effect. Your doctor may want to check your PT regularly. |

| Drug Interaction | Rating* | Potential Effects/Recommendations |
|---|---|---|
| Coumadin/Noroxin | D | Coumadin may have a more potent effect. Your doctor may want to check your PT while you are taking Noroxin. |
| Coumadin/Prilosec | D | Coumadin may have a slightly more potent effect. Your doctor may want to check your PT regularly. |
| Coumadin/Questran | A | Coumadin may be less effective. Take Coumadin at least three hours before or after Questran. Your doctor may want to check your PT frequently, or may replace Questran with a different cholesterol-lowering medication. |
| Coumadin/Quinidine | B | Although rare, Coumadin may have a more potent effect. Your doctor may want to check your PT regularly. |
| Coumadin/Quinine (in Q-Vel, Legatrin) | B | Although rare, Coumadin may have a more potent effect. Check with your doctor before you take any nonprescription product that contains quinine. |
| Coumadin/ Sulfonamides | A | Coumadin may have a more potent effect. Your doctor may want to check your PT and may adjust your Coumadin dosage while you taking the antibiotic. |
| Coumadin/Tagamet | A | Coumadin may be more effective. Your doctor may want to check your PT when you start, stop, or change the dosage of Tagamet. |

* The rating indicates how harmful a drug interaction may be and how frequently it may occur.

"A" indicates a drug interaction that may cause serious harm and occurs frequently. "B" indicates a drug interaction that may cause serious harm but occurs less frequently. "C" indicates a drug interaction that is less harmful but occurs frequently. "D" indicates a drug interaction that is less harmful and occurs less frequently. See Key 9 for more information about the rating system.

# 20

## MEDICATIONS FOR BRONCHITIS AND ASTHMA

*Bronchitis* is a condition in which the airways of the lungs are inflamed and swollen. Swelling narrows the airways, making it difficult for air to pass through. In addition, mucus secretions begin to fill the airways, creating an obstruction.

*Asthma* is a condition in which spasms occur in the airways to the lungs, resulting in constriction (closing). Wheezing, the high-pitched sound characteristic of asthma and bronchitis, is the result of air passing quickly through a narrow opening.

### The Medications

Five categories of medications are used to improve breathing in bronchitis or asthma:
1. sympathomimetics: *Alupent, Brethine, Bronkaid Mist, Duo-Medihaler, Isuprel, Maxair, Metaprel, Primatene Mist, Proventil, Tornalate,* and *Ventolin.*
2. xanthines: *aminophylline, Choledyl, Lufyllin,* and *theophylline.*
3. anticholinergic inhaler: *Atrovent.*
4. corticosteroids: *AeroBid, Azmacort, Beclovent,* and *Decadron.* (Ingested corticosteroids are discussed in Key 29.)
5. mucolytic expectorants: *Organidin, potassium iodide,* and *SSKI.*

Drug treatment for bronchitis or asthma may include one or more of these categories. The sympathomimetics, xanthines, and Atrovent inhaler all act to dilate (open) the bronchial

68

airways. The corticosteroids reduce swelling and inflammation. Mucolytic expectorants bring up mucus.

Many of these medications are available as inhalers, which is desirable because the drug is sprayed directly into the lungs rather ingested orally and traveling through the bloodstream to reach the lungs. Because the inhaled drug does not enter the bloodstream, side effects are minimal.

The most frequently prescribed xanthine is theophylline *(Bronkodyl, Elixophyllin, Quibron-T, Slo-bid Gyrocaps, Slo-Phyllin, T-Phyl, Theo-24, Theobid, Theo-Dur, Theolair, Uniphyl)*. It is available orally as a tablet, sustained-release tablet, capsule, sustained-release capsule, syrup, elixir, solution, and "sprinkle," in which the contents of a capsule are sprinkled on food and then eaten.

### Side Effects and Drug Interactions

#### Xanthines

Of the bronchial medications, the category that produces the most side effects is the xanthines. All of the drugs in the xanthine category are ingested orally and must therefore travel through the bloodstream to reach the lungs.

Theophylline dosing can be tricky. If the amount of theophylline in the bloodstream becomes too high, side effects, such as nausea, vomiting, headache, irritability, insomnia, and diarrhea, may occur. Other side effects involving the heart may also result if the amount of theophylline in the blood becomes extremely high. Conversely, if the amount of theophylline in the blood is too low, the drug may not be effective.

To prevent theophylline side effects or lack of effectiveness, your doctor may want to check your theophylline blood level (the amount of theophylline in the blood) on a regular basis. (This is especially true if you are taking other medications that may increase the potency or decrease the effectiveness of theophylline.) If the blood level results are too high or low, your doctor may adjust your dosage.

## Sympathomimetics

Sympathomimetics may aggravate certain conditions such as high blood pressure. Therefore, if you are taking a blood-pressure medication, check with your doctor before using nonprescription bronchoinhalers such as Bronkaid Mist or Primatene Mist. Inhalers such as these contain epinephrine, an ingredient that opposes the action of some blood-pressure medications, which results in increased blood pressure.

If you are taking a beta blocker such as Inderal and you develop shortness of breath or have difficulty breathing, tell your doctor immediately because these symptoms may be caused by the beta blocker. Do not use nonprescription bronchoinhalers to rectify the problem because they probably will not be effective. Some beta blockers oppose the action of epinephrine, thereby negating the beneficial effects of these bronchoinhalers. This is another example of a drug interaction caused by drug antagonism. (See Key 6, Drug Antagonism.)

### DRUG INTERACTION CHART: MEDICATIONS FOR BRONCHITIS AND ASTHMA

| Drug Interaction | Rating* | Potential Effects/Recommendations |
| --- | --- | --- |
| Brethine/Beta Blockers | C | Brethine may be less effective if you are taking a nonselective beta blocker. |
| Isuprel/Beta Blockers | A | Isuprel may not be effective if you are taking Inderal. Lopressor is less likely to interact; Normodyne (Trandate) has been shown not to interact. |
| Lufyllin/Benemid | B | Lufyllin may have a more potent action. Your doctor may want to check your Lufyllin blood level when you start or stop Benemid, or replace Lufyllin with theophylline, a medication that does not interact with Benemid. |
| Theophylline/ Barbiturates | C | Theophylline may be less effective. Your doctor may want to check your theophylline blood level when you start or stop the barbiturate. |

| Drug Interaction | Rating* | Potential Effects/Recommendations |
|---|---|---|
| Theophylline/Beta Blockers | A | Theophylline may have a more potent effect when combined with a non-selective beta blocker. Your doctor may adjust your theophylline dosage. |
| Theophylline/Calan | B | Theophylline may have a more potent effect. Your doctor may want to adjust your theophylline dosage. |
| Theopylline/Cardizem | D | Theophylline may be less effective. Your doctor may want to check your theophylline blood level periodically. |
| Theopylline/Charcoal | A | Theophylline may not be absorbed and may not be effective. Ask your pharmacist to recommend an intestinal gas medication that does not contain charcoal. |
| Theophylline/Cipro | A | Theophylline may have a more potent effect, especially in older people. Your doctor may want to check your theophylline blood level while you are taking Cipro. |
| Theophylline/Dilantin | C | Theophylline and Dilantin may both be less effective. Your doctor may adjust the dosages of both medications. Do not skip doses of either drug. |
| Theophylline/ Ephedrine | D | You may experience increased nervousness, insomnia, or stomach upset. If you do, contact your doctor. |
| Theophylline/ Erythromycin | A | Theophylline may have a more potent effect, and erythromycin may be less effective, after several days of combined use. Your doctor may adjust the dosages of both medications. |
| Theopylline/Food | C | The effectivness of some brands of theophylline may be changed if they are taken with a high-fat-content meal. Theo-24 and Uniphyl may exhibit a |

71

| Drug Interaction | Rating* | Potential Effects/Recommendations |
|---|---|---|
| | | more potent effect; Theolair and Theo-Dur Sprinkle may be less effective. (Theo-Dur Sprinkle will not be less effective if it is sprinkled on a spoonful of applesauce or pudding and taken one hour before or two hours after your meal.) The theophylline products that are not affected by food are Theo-Dur tablets, Slo-Bid Gyrocaps and Theobid. You may take these at any time. |
| Theophylline/ Isoniazid (INH) | C | Theophylline may have a more potent effect after several weeks of INH treatment. Your doctor may want to check your theophylline blood level regularly. |
| Theophylline/ Isoptin | B | Theophylline may have a more potent effect. Your doctor may want to adjust your theophylline dosage. |
| Theophylline/Lithium | C | See Key 24. |
| Theophylline/Mexitil | A | Theophylline may have a more potent effect. Your doctor may want to check your theophylline blood level frequently and may adjust your dosage. |
| Theopylline/Mintezol | B | Theophylline may have a more potent effect. Your doctor may want to check your theophylline blood level regularly. |
| Theophylline/Nizoral | D | Sustained-released forms of theophylline may not be completely absorbed, and theophylline may be less effective. Your doctor may adjust your theophylline dosage while you are taking Nizoral. |
| Theophylline/Noroxin | C | Theophylline may have a more potent effect. Your doctor may check your theophylline blood level while you are taking Noroxin. |

| Drug Interaction | Rating* | Potential Effects/Recommendations |
|---|---|---|
| Theophylline/ Prednisone | D | Theophylline may have a more potent effect. Your doctor may want to check your theophylline blood level periodically. |
| Theophylline/ Procardia | D | Although rare, theophylline may have a slightly more potent effect. |
| Theophylline/ Propylthiouricil (PTU) | C | The effectiveness of theophylline may change when you start or stop PTU. Your doctor may want to check your theophylline blood level regularly. (This drug interaction does not apply to you if you have been taking the same dose of PTU for years and are now starting theophylline.) |
| Theophylline/Rifampin | A | Theophylline may be less effective. Your doctor may adjust your dosage. Do not stop taking rifampin without your doctor's permission; doing so may cause theophylline's effect to be more potent and thereby lead to side effects. |
| Theophylline/Tagamet | A | Theophylline may have a more potent effect. Your doctor may check your theophylline blood level and may adjust your dosage. |
| Theophylline/Tapazole | C | The effectiveness of theophylline may change when you start or stop Tapazole. Your doctor may want to check your theophylline blood level regularly. (This drug interaction does not apply to you if you have been taking the same dose of Tapazole for years and are now starting theophylline.) |
| Theophylline/Tegretol | D | Theophylline may be less effective. Your doctor may want to check your theophylline blood level when you start or stop Tegretol. |

73

| Drug Interaction | Rating* | Potential Effects/Recommendations |
| --- | --- | --- |
| Theophylline/<br>Thyroid Hormones | C | The effectiveness of theophylline may change when you start or stop the thyroid medication. Your doctor may want to check your theophylline blood level regularly. (This drug interaction does not apply to you if you have been taking the same dose of thyroid hormone for years and are now starting theophylline.) |

* The rating indicates how harmful a drug interaction may be and how frequently it may occur.

"A" indicates a drug interaction that may cause serious harm and occurs frequently. "B" indicates a drug interaction that may cause serious harm but occurs less frequently. "C" indicates a drug interaction that is less harmful but occurs frequently. "D" indicates a drug interaction that is less harmful and occurs less frequently. See Key 9 for more information about the rating system.

# 21

# MEDICATIONS TO TREAT ANXIETY AND INSOMNIA

*Anxiety* is an unpleasant emotional state that may be described as a feeling of exaggerated nervousness, agitation, worry, and fearfulness caused by an unsettling event or the anticipation of an unsettling event (such as an illness in the family or marital problems). However, anxiety is not necessarily linked to an event—it can occur without an obvious cause.

*Insomnia* may be described as the inability to fall asleep or to stay asleep throughout the night. Insomnia may be caused by tension, stress, pain, discomfort, or traumatic event, but can occur even when none of these is present. Some forms of insomnia, in fact, such as early-morning awakening, occur quite commonly as we get older.

## The Medications

**Medications to treat anxiety** are as follows:

1. benzodiazepines: *Ativan, Centrax, diazepam, Librium, Paxipam, Serax, Tranxene, Valium,* and *Xanax.*
2. *meprobamate.*
3. *BuSpar.*
4. antihistamines: *Atarax* and *Vistaril,* discussed in Key 27.
5. tricyclic antidepressants (TCAs): *Adapin, doxepin, Sinequan,* discussed in Key 23.

**Medications to treat insomnia** are as follows:

1. benzodiazepines: *Dalmane, Doral, Halcion, ProSom,* and *Restoril.*
2. barbiturates: *Nembutal,* discussed in Key 22.
3. miscellaneous: *Noctec, Noludar,* and *Placidyl.*

# Side Effects and Drug Interactions

All of the anxiety and insomnia medications may cause some degree of dizziness, daytime sleepiness, weakness, reduced coordination, and slower reaction time. Therefore, if you are taking any of these medications, you should use caution if you have to drive your car or perform tasks that require alertness. (Older people may be especially susceptible to these side effects.)

If you take anxiety or insomnia medications with other medications that also cause drowsiness and dizziness, such as antihistamines, the combination may have an overwhelming effect (lack of coordination, intensified and extended sedation). Check with your doctor or pharmacist before combining your anxiety or insomnia medication with a nonprescription drug product. Remember that alcoholic beverages, even a single glass of wine, may have a similar effect on your medication.

In the drug interaction chart in this Key, you may notice that some benzodiazepines interact with Tagamet, Prilosec, and estrogens, while others (Ativan, Restoril and Serax) do not. The difference between the benzodiazepines that interact and those that do not has to do with the way they are metabolized (broken down) before being eliminated from the body. For example, Tagamet may decrease the metabolism and subsequent elimination of Xanax from the body if the two drugs are taken together. Because Xanax has not been completely metabolized, it is still available in the bloodstream to produce its action, resulting in a more potent effect. However, Tagamet does not affect Ativan's potency because Ativan is metabolized differently from Xanax.

# DRUG INTERACTION CHART:
## MEDICATIONS TO TREAT ANXIETY AND INSOMNIA

| Drug Interaction | Rating* | Potential Effects/Recommendations |
| --- | --- | --- |
| Benzodiazepines/ Alcohol | A | You may become oversedated and experience severe loss of coordination. Ask your doctor whether you may drink alcoholic beverages with your benzodiazepine and, if so, what quantity is safe. |
| Benzodiazepines/ Benemid | D | The benzodiazepine may have a more prolonged action. Your doctor may adjust your benzodiazepine dosage. |
| Benzodiazepines/ Digoxin | B | See Key 17, "Digoxin/Valium or Xanax." |
| Benzodiazepines/ Estrogens | D | Some benzodiazepines may have a more potent effect; others (Ativan, Serax, and Restoril) may be less effective. Your doctor may adjust your benzodiazepine dosage. |
| Benzodiazepines/ Isoniazid (INH) | D | Valium or Halcion may have a more potent effect. Your doctor may adjust your benzodiazepine dosage. |
| Benzodiazepines/ Prilosec | D | Some benzodiazepines may have a more potent effect. Your doctor may adjust your benzodiazepine dosage. (Ativan, Restoril, and Serax do not interact with Prilosec.) |
| Benzodiazepines/ Rifampin | D | Some benzodiazepines, such as Valium, Tranxene, Centrax, and Paxipam, may be less effective. Your doctor may adjust your benzodiazepine dosage. |
| Benzodiazepines/ Tagamet | C | The benzodiazepine may have a more potent effect. Your doctor may adjust the benzodiazepine dosage while you take Tagamet. (Ativan, Restoril, and Serax do not interact). |

| Drug Interaction | Rating* | Potential Effects/Recommendations |
|---|---|---|
| BuSpar/Prozac | D | BuSpar may be less effective. Your doctor may adjust your BuSpar dosage. |
| Halcion/Erythromycin | C | Halcion may have a more potent effect after you have taken both drugs for several days. If you feel sleepy during the daytime, tell your doctor. |
| Meprobamate/Alcohol | A | You may become excessively drowsy and dizzy. Avoid large amounts of alcohol. Ask your doctor whether you may drink alcholic beverages and, if so, what quantity is safe. |
| Noctec/Alcohol | A | You may become oversedated and experience severe loss of coordination. Although rare, facial flushing may occur. Ask your doctor whether you may drink alcoholic beverages and, if so, what quantity is safe. |
| Sleep Medications/ Antihistamines | A | You may feel oversedated the next morning. Do not combine a sleep medication with an antihistamine without first asking your doctor. |

* The rating indicates how harmful a drug interaction may be and how frequently it may occur.

   "A" indicates a drug interaction that may cause serious harm and occurs frequently. "B" indicates a drug interaction that may cause serious harm but occurs less frequently. "C" indicates a drug interaction that is less harmful but occurs frequently. "D" indicates a drug interaction that is less harmful and occurs less frequently. See Key 9 for more information about the rating system.

# 22

## BARBITURATES—DRUGS WITH MANY USES

Years ago, *barbiturates* were often prescribed as sedatives and as sleeping pills, but this is not true anymore. Nowadays, the treatment of choice for sedation and insomnia is a selection from the menu of the benzodiazepine classification of drugs.

Phenobarbital is a barbiturate prescribed primarily to control seizures in people who have epilepsy. The barbiturate butalbital is often combined with aspirin (Fioricet) or acetaminophen (Fiorinal) to relieve moderately severe headaches. Barbiturates such as pentobarbital and Amytal are frequently used in hospitals before surgery or other procedures that require anesthesia.

### The Medications

The following orally dosed medications are classified as barbiturates: *Amytal, butalbital, Butisol Sodium, Gemonil, Mebaral, Nembutal, pentobarbital, phenobarbital,* and *Seconal. Tuinal* is a drug product that contains two barbiturates, Amytal and Seconal.

Headache medications such as *Fioricet, Esgic, Fiorinal,* and *Phrenilin* all contain the barbiturate butalbital.

*Mysoline,* a medication for epilepsy, is not really a barbiturate itself. Once absorbed into the bloodsteam, however, Mysoline is broken down into other components, one of which is phenobarbital.

### Side Effects and Drug Interactions

All of the barbiturates produce similar side effects—excessive sleepiness or a "hangover" feeling is the most common. Lethargy, dizziness, lack of coordination, and confusion may become more pronounced with higher doses. Barbiturate overdose can be fatal because the drug can alter heart, lung, and brain function.

Barbiturates can change the effectiveness of other medications by increasing the speed at which they are metabolized. If a drug is broken down into its inactive form earlier than intended, the drug cannot produce its usual action completely and may therefore be less effective. In most cases, the action of the barbiturate is not affected.

Combining barbiturates with other drugs that cause drowsiness and dizziness can be dangerous because the total effect of the combined medications may be overwhelmingly potent and may result in unwanted (and sometimes serious) side effects.

Finally, although alcohol is not a medication, it cannot be overlooked as a drug that can and does interact with barbiturates. If you are taking a barbiturate and planning to go to a party at which alcoholic beverages will be served, you may want to ask your doctor whether you may have a drink or two. The answer will probably depend on many factors individual to you that only your doctor can consider.

### DRUG INTERACTION CHART:
### BARBITURATES—DRUGS WITH MANY USES

| Drug Interaction | Rating* | Potential Effects/Recommendations |
| --- | --- | --- |
| Barbiturates/Alcohol | A | Sudden consumption of large amounts of alcohol may increase the potency and effects of barbiturates. Therefore, you may become oversedated and may experience severe loss of coordination. |
| Barbiturates/ Anticoagulants | A | See Key 19. |
| Barbiturates/ Beta Blockers | C | See Key 14. |
| Barbiturates/ Butazolidin | D | See Key 26. |

| Drug Interaction | Rating* | Potential Effects/Recommendations |
|---|---|---|
| Barbiturates/Charcoal | C | The barbiturate may not be fully absorbed and therefore may be less effective. Ask your pharmacist to help you select an intestinal gas medication that does not contain charcoal. |
| Barbiturates/ Corticosteroids | C | See Key 29. |
| Barbiturates/Darvon or Darvocet-N | D | The barbiturate may have a more potent effect. If you are taking Darvon or Darvocet-N, ask your doctor whether you may also take your barbiturate medication. |
| Barbiturates/Quinidine | A | See Key 16. |
| Barbiturates/TCAs | C | See Key 23. |
| Barbiturates/ Theophylline | C | See Key 20. |
| Barbiturates/Thorazine | D | See Key 24. |
| Mysoline/Alcohol | A | Sudden consumption of large amounts of alcohol may increase the potency and effects of barbiturates. Therefore, you may become oversedated and may experience severe loss of coordination. |
| Mysoline/ Anticoagulants | A | See Key 19. |
| Mysoline/ Corticosteroids | C | See Key 29. |
| Mysoline/Depakene or Depakote | A | Mysoline may have a more potent effect. Your doctor may adjust the dosage of Mysoline when Depakene is added to your drug therapy. |
| Mysoline/Diamox | B | Mysoline may be less effective. Your doctor may adjust the dosage of Mysoline. |
| Mysoline/Dilantin | C | Mysoline may have a more potent effect. Your doctor may adjust the dosage of Mysoline when Dilantin is added to your drug therapy. |

81

| Drug Interaction | Rating* | Potential Effects/Recommendations |
|---|---|---|
| Mysoline/Fulvicin | D | See Key 32. |
| Mysoline/Isoniazid (INH) | D | Mysoline may have a more potent effect. Your doctor may want to check your Mysoline dosage while you are taking INH. |
| Mysoline/Quinidine | A | See Key 16. |
| Mysoline/Tegretol | C | Mysoline may be less effective; Tegretol may have a more potent effect. Your doctor may want to check the effects of both medications regularly. |
| Phenobarbital/Calan | A | See Key 15, "CCBs/Phenobarbital." |
| Phenobarbital/ Depakene or Depakote | A | Phenobarbital may have a more potent effect. Your doctor may want to check your phenobarbital blood levels regularly. |
| Phenobarbital/Fulvicin | D | See Key 32. |
| Phenobarbital/Haldol | C | See Key 24. |
| Phenobarbital/Norpace | A | See Key 16. |
| Phenobarbital/ Procardia | A | See Key 15, "CCBs/Phenobarbital." |
| Phenobarbital/Tegretol | C | See Key 30. |

* The rating indicates how harmful a drug interaction may be and how frequently it may occur.

"A" indicates a drug interaction that may cause serious harm and occurs frequently. "B" indicates a drug interaction that may cause serious harm but occurs less frequently. "C" indicates a drug interaction that is less harmful but occurs frequently. "D" indicates a drug interaction that is less harmful and occurs less frequently. See Key 9 for more information about the rating system.

# 23

# MEDICATIONS TO TREAT DEPRESSION

*Depression* may be described as an ongoing mood of deep sadness, emptiness, dejection, and feeling of failure. Depression may result from a series of stressful events or the occurrence of a single traumatic happening, such as the breakup of a relationship, the loss of a job, or the death of a loved one.

Everyone may experience feelings of depression from time to time, but most people eventually feel better. Others, however, cannot pull themselves out of a constantly depressed mood. They feel unmotivated and have trouble concentrating on their work or hobbies.

People who are diagnosed with depression may benefit from antidepressants (medications for depression) which help them to concentrate better, increase their motivation, and improve their ability to deal with stressful situations.

## The Medications

The antidepressants may be divided into three categories:
1. tricyclic antidepressants (TCAs): *Adapin, Anafranil, Asendin, amitriptyline, Aventyl, desipramine, doxepin, Elavil, Endep, imipramine, Norpramin, nortriptyline, Pamelor, Pertofrane, Sinequan, Surmontil, Tofranil, trazodone,* and *Vivactil.*
2. monoamine oxidase inhibitors (MAOIs): *Marplan, Nardil,* and *Parnate.*
3. miscellaneous antidepressants: *Desyrel, Ludiomil, Prozac,* and *Wellbutrin.*

## Side Effects and Drug Interactions

All of the medications in the TCA category are chemically related to each other. Because they are so similar, they all tend to produce similar side effects and also interact in the same way with other medications. The same is true of the MAOI category of drugs.

### Tricyclic Antidepressants (TCAs)

The most common side effects of the TCAs are sedation, dizziness, dry mouth, constipation, and confusion (which is more likely occur in older people). In older men, a decreased ability to urinate is also quite common. When the TCA is combined with other medications that may cause the antidepressant to have a more potent effect, all of the above side effects may become worse. Other side effects such as facial flushing, agitation, increased drowsiness, and heart abnormalities, may also occur.

Many nonprescription drug products (for example, cough/cold/allergy medications) contain ingredients that may cause drowsiness, dizziness, difficult urination, and dry mouth. When such a product is combined with a TCA, these side effects not only are more likely to occur but also may be more pronounced. Always check with your doctor or pharmacist before taking a nonprescription drug product with your TCA.

### Monoamine Oxidase Inhibitors (MAOIs)

The MAOIs most often interact with other medications to produce two kinds of reactions:

1. The MAOI may have a more potent effect and produce such symptoms as dizziness, nausea, excitability, muscle weakness, and facial flushing.
2. The interaction may result in headache (which can be severe), and a sudden increase in blood pressure.

The second kind of reaction is more likely to occur when MAOIs are combined with decongestants, diet aids that contain phenylpropranolamine (PPA), or tyramine, an amino acid (protein) found in some foods and alcoholic beverages. The reaction caused by the combination of MAOIs and tyramine can be severe, so your doctor will probably give you a list of foods to avoid if you are taking a MAOI. Aged cheeses, fermented meats (salami, bologna, pepperoni), pickled herring and red wine are among the worst offenders! For a more complete list of foods and beverages that contain tyramine, see Key 44.

## DRUG INTERACTION CHART:
## MEDICATIONS TO TREAT DEPRESSION

| Drug Interaction | Rating* | Potential Effects/Recommendations |
|---|---|---|
| Desyrel/Prozac | D | Desyrel may have a more potent effect. Your doctor may adjust your Desyrel dosage. |
| MAOIs/Alcohol | A | Some alcoholic beverages contain large amounts of tyramine, an ingredient that can trigger sudden high blood pressure and other side effects in persons taking MAOIs. Ask your doctor whether you may drink alcoholic beverages with your medication and, if so, how much is safe. Avoid red wines (especially Chianti) and imported beers because these beverages contain large amounts of tyramine. |
| MAOIs/Decongestants | A | Combining MAOIs and decongestants such as Sudafed, ephedrine, phenylphrine, and phenylpropanolamine (PPA) may cause headache and increased blood pressure that can lead to other side effects. Do not take a decongestant without first asking your doctor. Beware—many cold/allergy products contain decongestants. Ask your pharmacist to help you select a product that does not contain a decongestant. |
| MAOIs/Demerol | A | You may experience side effects such as sweating, excitability, and increased blood pressure. If you experience these symptoms, contact your doctor. |

| Drug Interaction | Rating* | Potential Effects/Recommendations |
|---|---|---|
| MAOIs/Diet Aids | A | Many nonprescription diet aids contain phenylpropanolamine (PPA), an ingredient that can cause headache and increased blood pressure. Check with your doctor before you start your diet. |
| MAOIs/Foods | A | You may experience headache and sudden increased blood pressure if you eat foods that contain large amounts of tyramine while you are being treated with a MAOI. Foods that are fermented, aged, or overripe tend to be high in tyramine content. See Key 44 for a list of foods that should not be eaten with MAOIs. |
| MAOIs/Levodopa | A | Combining MAOIs, except Elderpryl, with levodopa can cause light-headedness, flushing of the face, pounding of the heart, and increased blood pressure. People who are taking Sinemet are less likely to experience these side effects. |
| MAOIs/Neo-Synephrine Nasal Spray | C | See Key 40. |
| MAOIs/Prozac | A | You may experience side effects such as shivering, restlessness, nausea, or increased muscle tone. If these side effects occur, contact your doctor. |
| MAOIs/Sulfonamides | B | Although side effects are uncommon with this combination, you could experience dizziness, weakness, muscle pain and ringing in the ears. If you have these symptoms, contact your doctor. |
| MAOIs/TCAs | B | Although many people combine MAOIs and TCAs without any ill effect, side effects, such as excitability, facial flushing, high body temperature, and mood changes can occur. If you experience any of these symptoms, contact your doctor. |
| Prozac/BuSpar | D | See Key 21. |

| Drug Interaction | Rating* | Potential Effects/Recommendations |
|---|---|---|
| TCAs/Alcohol | A | See Key 43. |
| TCAs/Antispasmodics | B | See Key 11. |
| TCAs/Barbiturates | C | The TCA may be less effective. Your doctor may adjust your TCA dosage. |
| TCAs/Bronkaid Mist | B | See Key 42. |
| TCAs/Decongestants | A | Cold/allergy products that contain phenylephrine may increase the risk of abnormal heartbeat. Check with your doctor before taking a nonprescription medication that contains a decongestant. |
| TCAs/Diabetes Medicines | D | See Key 28. |
| TCAs/Ismelin | A | See Key 12. |
| TCAs/Levodopa | D | See Key 34. |
| TCAs/Lithium | D | The TCA may have a more potent effect. Your doctor may adjust your TCA dosage. |
| TCAs/Neo-Synephrine Nasal Spray | B | Excessive doses of Neo-Synephrine may lead to a sudden increase in blood pressure. Ask your doctor whether you may use Neo-Synephrine with your TCA. |
| TCAs/Phenothiazines | D | The TCA may have a more potent effect. Your doctor may adjust your TCA dosage. |
| TCAs/Primatene Mist | B | See Key 42. |
| TCAs/Prozac | A | The TCA may have a more potent effect. This interaction may occur several weeks after you have begun to take these medications together. See your doctor regularly so that your drug treatment can be evaluated. |
| TCAs/Quinidine | A | The TCA may have a more potent effect. Your doctor will probably want to examine you regularly to check the dosage of your TCA. |

87

| Drug Interaction | Rating* | Potential Effects/Recommendations |
|---|---|---|
| TCAs/Tagamet | A | The TCA may have a more potent effect. Your doctor may want to check your TCA blood level regularly and may adjust the dosage. |
| Tofranil/Beta Blockers | B | Tofranil may have a more potent effect when combined with Normodyne (Trandate). Your doctor may want to examine you regularly and may adjust your Tofranil dosage. |

* The rating indicates how harmful a drug interaction may be and how frequently it may occur.

"A" indicates a drug interaction that may cause serious harm and occurs frequently. "B" indicates a drug interaction that may cause serious harm but occurs less frequently. "C" indicates a drug interaction that is less harmful but occurs frequently. "D" indicates a drug interaction that is less harmful and occurs less frequently. See Key 9 for more information about the rating system.

# 24

## MEDICATIONS FOR PSYCHIATRIC DISORDERS

The term *psychiatric disorders* encompasses several types of mental illnesses in which a variety of symptoms may occur, such as hysteria, paranoia, compulsive or obsessive behavior, exaggerated mood swings (manic-depression, known to psychiatrists as "bipolar disorder"), overaggresive behavior, or the inability to deal with reality (also known as "psychosis").

Treatment usually involves sessions with a psychiatrist, who will diagnose which type of mental illness the person is suffering from. Medications may or may not be part of the treatment.

### The Medications

The antipsychotic medications include the following:
1. phenothiazines: *chlorpromazine, Compazine, Mellaril, prochlorperazine, Prolixin, Serentil, Stelazine, Sparine, Thorazine, thoridazine, Tindal, Trilafon*, and *Vesprin*.
2. miscellaneous antipsychotic medications: *Clozaril, Eskalith, Haldol, haloperidol, lithium, Lithobid, Lithotab, Loxitane, Moban, Navane*, and *Orap*.

### Side Effects and Drug Interactions

**Phenothiazines**

One of the most common side effects of the phenothiazines is drowsiness; use caution if you drive your car or do other tasks that require alertness. Also, the phenothiazines may make you more susceptible to sunburn, so be sure to apply a sunscreen if you plan to be in the sun for an extended period of time.

After a phenothiazine has been taken for several months or years, other side effects such as jaundice, muscle tremors, or involuntary muscle movements of the mouth, jaw, and face are more likely to occur.

The phenothiazines are chemically similar to antihistamines, so do not combine these two classes of drugs without first checking with your doctor. Beware: many nonprescription drug products (for example, sleeping aids and motion sickness tablets) contain antihistamines. Ask your pharmacist to help you select over-the-counter products that will not interact with your phenothiazine.

## Miscellaneous Antipsychotic Medications

Lithium carbonate (Eskalith, Lithobid, Lithotab) is a medication prescribed to treat manic-depressive illness, a condition in which exaggerated mood swings occur. Although this drug truly deserves to be recognized as a "wonder drug" because it allows manic-depressives to live nearly normal lives, lithium can be dangerous.

The major concern about lithium is that the correct dosage is not too different from the harmful or ineffective dosage. In other words, there's not much margin for error with lithium. If the dosage is too high, you may experience such side effects as nausea, vomiting, diarrhea, muscle weakness, and lack of coordination. If the dosage is too low, the medication may become less effective or even ineffective.

Activities that cause you to perspire—playing tennis or exercising in the hot sun, for example—may also increase the potency of lithium. Therefore you should check with your doctor before engaging in any rigorous activity that may cause perspiration.

Because lithium dosing is so critical, your doctor may want to check your lithium blood level (the amount of lithium in your blood) regularly. In that way, if the blood level is too high or too low, your doctor can adjust your dosage.

Haldol, when taken over long periods of time, may cause muscle tremors and involuntary muscle movements of the mouth, jaw, and face. When Haldol is combined with other medications that increase its potency, excessive sedation and severe tremor may occur. On the other hand, drug interactions that cause Haldol to lose effectiveness may result in increased symptoms related to the psychiatric illness.

## DRUG INTERACTION CHART:
## MEDICATIONS FOR PSYCHIATRIC DISORDERS

| Drug Interaction | Rating* | Potential Effects/Recommendations |
|---|---|---|
| Haldol/Aldomet | B | You may experience mood changes or feel irritable or disoriented. If you do, contact your doctor. You may need a Haldol dosage adjustment. |
| Haldol/Antispasmodics Medications | A | Haldol may be less effective; your symptoms may worsen. Haldol side effects, such as involuntary muscle movements, can occur. If you experience these effects, contact your doctor. |
| Haldol/Dilantin | D | Haldol may be less effective. Your doctor may want to examine you regularly to check for medication effectiveness. |
| Haldol/Inderal | B | Both drugs may have more potent effect. Your doctor may adjust the dosages of both medications. |
| Haldol/Ismelin | D | See Key 12. |
| Haldol/Phenobarbital | C | Haldol may be less effective. Your doctor may want to examine you regularly and may adjust your Haldol dosage. |
| Haldol/Prozac | B | You may experience uncoordinated body movements or tremors. If you do, contact your doctor. Your doctor may want to examine you regularly to check for these kinds of side effects. |

91

| Drug Interaction | Rating* | Potential Effects/Recommendations |
| --- | --- | --- |
| Haldol/Rifampin | D | Haldol may be less effective. Your doctor may adjust the dosage while you are taking rifampin. |
| Haldol/Tegretol | C | Haldol may be less effective. Your doctor may adjust your Haldol dosage. |
| Lithium/Aldactone | D | Lithium may have a slightly more potent effect. Your doctor may want to check your lithium blood level regularly. |
| Lithium/Aldomet | B | Lithium may have a more potent effect. Your doctor may check your lithium blood level regularly and may adjust your dosage. |
| Lithium/Beta Blockers | D | Lithium may have a slightly more potent effect. Your doctor may want to check your lithium blood level regularly. |
| Lithium/Bumex | B | Lithium may have a more potent effect. Your doctor may want to check your lithium blood level when you start or stop Bumex. |
| Lithium/CCBs | A | Calan (Isoptin) or Cardizem combined with lithium may cause such symptoms as nausea, vomiting, weakness, tremor, and ringing in the ears. If you experience these symptoms, contact your doctor *immediately*. |
| Lithium/Feldene | D | Although rare, lithium may have a more potent effect. Your doctor may want to check your lithium blood level when you start or stop Feldene. |
| Lithium/Haldol | A | Although these medications are used together, large doses of both may cause side effects. If you feel feverish, lethargic, and disoriented, contact your doctor. |
| Lithium/Ibuprofen | C | Lithium may have a more potent effect if you are taking ibuprofen every day. Check with your doctor before taking nonprescription ibuprofen with lithium. |

| Drug Interaction | Rating* | Potential Effects/Recommendations |
|---|---|---|
| Lithium/Indocin | C | Lithium may have a more potent effect. Your doctor may want to check your lithium blood level when you start or stop Indocin. |
| Lithium/Lasix | D | Lithium may have a more potent effect. Your doctor may want to check your lithium blood level when you start or stop Lasix. |
| Lithium/Prozac | D | Lithium may have a more potent effect. Your doctor may want to check your lithium blood level regularly. |
| Lithium/Salt (Sodium Chloride) | C | Either an *excessive amount* of table salt or a *salt-restricted diet* can change the effectiveness of lithium. Be consistent with your salt intake. |
| Lithium/Tegretol | B | Although this combination may not be a common one, lithium side effects (muscle weakness, tremor, loss of coordination, and lethargy) can occur. Because these side effects may occur even when the lithium blood level is in the normal range, your doctor may want to examine you frequently. |
| Lithium/Theophylline | C | Lithium may be less effective. Your doctor may want to check your lithium blood level frequently. Do not skip doses of either medication. |
| Lithium/Thiazides | A | Lithium may have a more potent effect. If you experience side effects such as drowsiness, loss of coordination, nausea, vomiting, or diarrhea, contact your doctor *immediately*. |
| Lithium/Thorazine | C | The effectiveness of both medications may change. Your doctor may want to examine you regularly to check for medication side effects. |
| Loxitane/Dilantin | D | See Key 30. |
| Navane/Ismelin | D | See Key 12. |

| Drug Interaction | Rating* | Potential Effects/Recommendations |
|---|---|---|
| Phenothiazines/ Alcohol | A | You may feel excessively drowsy or dizzy and experience loss of coordination, tremors, or involuntary muscle movements. Ask your doctor whether you may drink alcoholic beverages with your phenothiazine and if so, what quantity is safe. |
| Phenothiazines/ Antihistamines | A | *Drug duplication:* the phenothiazines are chemically similar to antihistamines and should not be taken with them unless your doctor instructs you to do so. |
| Phenothiazines/ Antispasmodics | D | The phenothiazine may be less effective. Your doctor may want to examine you regularly and may adjust your dosage. |
| Phenothiazines/ Charcoal | C | Phenothiazines may not be fully absorbed and may therefore be less effective. Ask your pharmacist to help you select an intestinal gas medication that does not contain charcoal. |
| Phenothiazines/ Dilantin | D | See Key 30. |
| Phenothiazines/ Kaopectate | D | Phenothiazines may be less effective. Take the phenothiazine one hour before or two hours after Kaopectate. |
| Phenothiazines/ Lithium | B | You may feel disoriented, or involuntary muscle movements may occur. If so, contact your doctor. |
| Phenothiazines/ Norflex or Norgesic | C | The phenothiazine may be less effective. Also, you may experience side effects such as dry mouth, blurred vision, or dizziness. Your doctor may want to examine you regularly to check the side effects and dosages of your medications. |
| Phenothiazines/TCAs | D | See Key 23. |
| Thorazine/Antacids | D | Thorazine may not be completely absorbed. Take the antacid one hour before or two hours after Thorazine. |

| Drug Interaction | Rating* | Potential Effects/Recommendations |
|---|---|---|
| Thorazine/Barbiturates | D | Thorazine may be less effective. Your doctor may want to examine you regularly to check your medication therapy. |
| Thorazine/Capoten | B | See Key 12, "ACE Inhibitors (Capoten)/ Thorazine." |
| Thorazine/Demerol | A | You may feel excessively drowsy, faint and dizzy. Use caution if you must do tasks that require mental alertness, such as driving. |
| Thorazine/Depakene or Depakote | C | See Key 30. |
| Thorazine/Inderal | D | Both drugs may have more potent effects. Your doctor may adjust the dosages of both medications. |
| Thorazine/Ismelin | A | See Key 12. |

* The rating indicates how harmful a drug interaction may be and how frequently it may occur.

"A" indicates a drug interaction that may cause serious harm and occurs frequently. "B" indicates a drug interaction that may cause serious harm but occurs less frequently. "C" indicates a drug interaction that is less harmful but occurs frequently. "D" indicates a drug interaction that is less harmful and occurs less frequently. See Key 9 for more information about the rating system.

# 25

# MEDICATIONS FOR NAUSEA/ VOMITING/DIZZINESS/ MOTION SICKNESS

*Nausea* and *vomiting* need no description—unfortunately, we've all experienced these symptoms. The most difficult part about treating nausea and vomiting is determining their cause. The problem may be a common stomach virus, a more complex or serious disease, or even the medications the person is taking.

*Dizziness* (inability to maintain balance) is another symptom that commonly occurs with many illnesses and also as a side effect of many medications. A more serious kind of dizziness, *vertigo*, is caused by a disturbance in the inner ear that ultimately affects equilibrium. People who have experienced vertigo may describe it as a spinning sensation—either they are spinning around, or the room is spinning around them.

*Motion sickness* is caused by repetitive movements, such as the swaying motion of a boat or the up and down motion of a jet plane. Symptoms include sweating, skin pallor, nausea, and vomiting.

Determining the cause of the symptoms is very important because each illness may require a different kind of treatment.

### The Medications

Medications prescribed to relieve nausea and vomiting are as follows:

1. phenothiazines: *Compazine, Phenergan, Thorazine,* and *Torecan,* which are all available both as oral tablets and capsules and as rectal suppositories.

2. *Tigan*, which is also available as an oral capsule and a rectal suppository.

To relieve severe nausea and vomiting, rectal suppositories are often prescribed instead of tablets or capsules taken by mouth (orally). Oral medications can lose effectiveness if they are vomited before they have been completely absorbed, whereas the absorption of a suppository is not affected by vomiting.

The most commonly prescribed medication to treat vertigo is *Antivert (meclizine)*.

Medications prescribed to prevent motion sickness are as follows:

1. antihistamines: *Antivert, Benadryl, diphenhydramine,* and *meclizine*.
2. *Transderm Scōp*, a patch that is applied in back of the ear.

### Side Effects and Drug Interactions

The most frequent side effect of all of the medications listed above is drowsiness. Other side effects that may occur are dry mouth and blurred vision. You may be wondering why there aren't as many drug interactions listed for the phenothiazines in this Key, as compared to those in Key 24 (Medications for Psychiatric Disorders). The reason is that phenothiazines are usually taken on a temporary basis to treat nausea and vomiting, whereas the phenothiazines are taken over extended periods of time for psychiatric disorders.

The phenothiazines, Antivert, and the antihistamines are all chemically similar. Therefore, you should not take any of these medications with a nonprescription allergy, cough, or cold product that contains antihistamines. In addition, they should not be taken with a nonprescription sleep aid because it, too, contains an antihistamine. In the drug interaction chart for this Key, you will see these drug interactions marked *Drug duplication*. Your pharmacist can help you select nonprescription drug products that will not interact with your motion sickness or nausea/vomiting medication.

97

Is it safe to drink alcoholic beverages with any of these medications? That's a question you'll have to ask your doctor because the answer may be different for different people. Any of these medications combined with alcohol may result in extreme drowsiness and increased lack of coordination.

## DRUG INTERACTION CHART:
## MEDICATIONS FOR NAUSEA/VOMITING/DIZZINESS/MOTION SICKNESS

| Drug Interaction | Rating* | Potential Effects/Recommendations |
| --- | --- | --- |
| Compazine/ Antihistamines | A | *Drug duplication:* Compazine is chemically similar to the antihistamines. Check with your doctor before taking these medications together. |
| Compazine/ Nonprescription Sleep Aids | A | *Drug duplication:* Compazine is chemically similar to nonprescription sleep aids. Check with your doctor before taking these medications together. |
| Phenergan/ Antihistamines | A | *Drug duplication:* Phenergan is chemically similar to the antihistamines. Check with your doctor before taking these medications together. |
| Phenergan/Lithium | B | You may eel disoriented or may experience involuntary muscle movements. If these symptoms occur, contact your doctor *immediately*. |
| Phenergan/ Nonprescription Sleep Aids | A | *Drug duplication:* Phenergan is chemically similar to nonprescription sleep aids. Check with your doctor before taking these medications together. |
| Thorazine/ Antihistamines | A | *Drug duplication:* Thorazine is chemically similar to the antihistamines. Check with your doctor before taking these medications together. |

| Drug Interaction | Rating* | Potential Effects/Recommendations |
|---|---|---|
| Thorazine/ Nonprescription Sleep Aids | A | *Drug duplication:* Thorazine is chemically similar to nonprescription sleep aids. Check with your doctor before taking these medications together. |
| Thorazine/Demerol | A | You may feel drowsy, dizzy, or faint. Do not take this combination without first asking your doctor. |
| Transderm Scōp/ Alcohol | A | This combination is likely to occur if you take a cruise or fly in an airplane. Drinking alcoholic beverages while using the Transderm Scōp patch may lead to excessive drowsiness, dizziness, blurred vision, and dry mouth. Ask your doctor whether you may drink alcoholic beverages while using the patch and, if so, what quantity is safe. |
| Transderm Scōp/ Antihistamines | A | Dizziness, drowsiness, blurred vision, and dry mouth may occur when these medications are combined. Check with your doctor before taking antihistamines with Transderm Scōp. |

\* The rating indicates how harmful a drug interaction may be and how frequently it may occur.

"A" indicates a drug interaction that may cause serious harm and occurs frequently. "B" indicates a drug interaction that may cause serious harm but occurs less frequently. "C" indicates a drug interaction that is less harmful but occurs frequently. "D" indicates a drug interaction that is less harmful and occurs less frequently. See Key 9 for more information about the rating system.

# 26

## PAIN RELIEVERS/MUSCLE RELAXANTS/MIGRAINE HEADACHE PRODUCTS

*Pain* is the number one reason that people seek medical treatment. The causes of pain are numerous, and many categories of drugs (and medications) are available for treatment. Mild pain can usually be relieved by taking nonprescription acetaminophen, aspirin, or ibuprofen. Moderate pain may require a nonsteroidal anti-inflammatory drug (NSAID; see below), and severe pain may call for a narcotic pain reliever. Some drug products, such as Tylenol with Codeine, contain pain relievers from two or more categories.

The medication that your doctor prescribes for you will depend on the severity of the pain and the type of pain you have (what it is caused by). For example, aspirin or a NSAID is more effective than acetaminophen in relieving arthritis pain because acetaminophen does not reduce inflammation as aspirin and the NSAID do. Although all these drugs relieve pain, the added effect of reducing inflammation makes aspirin or ibuprofen a better choice than acetaminophen for treating arthritis pain.

### The Medications

The pain medications are divided into seven categories:
1. nonnarcotic pain relievers
    a. acetaminophen: *Tylenol* and numerous other brands.
    b. salicylates: *Arthropan, aspirin, Ben-Gay, Disalcid, Doan's Pills, Dolobid, Icy-Hot, sodium salicylate, Trilisate, Uracel,* and other medications that contain salicylates.

2. narcotic pain relievers: *Anexia, codeine, Darvon, Darvocet-N, Demerol, Dilaudid, Hydrocet, Levo-Dromoran, Lortab, methadone, morphine, Paregoric, Percocet, Percodan, Synalgos DC, Talacen, Talwin NX, Tylox, Vicodin,* and *Wygesic.*
3. nonsteroidal anti-inflammatory drugs (NSAIDs): *Anaprox, Ansaid, Clinoril, Feldene, ibuprofen, Indocin, indomethacin, Meclomen, Motrin, Nalfon, Naprosyn, Orudis, Rufen, Tolectin,* and *Voltaren.*
4. muscle relaxants: *carisoprodol, cyclobenzaprine, Dantrium, Flexeril, Lioresal, methocarbamol, Norflex, Parafon Forte DSC, Paraflex, Robaxin, Skelaxin, Soma,* and *Valium.*
5. gout medications: *Allopurinol, Anturane, Benemid,* and *Zyloprim.*
6. rheumatoid arthritis medications: *Butazolidin, methotrexate,* and *Ridaura.*
7. *ergotamine* contained in *Cafergot, Ergomar, Ergostat,* and *Wigraine.* (See Migraine Headache Medications in the Drug and Interaction table.)

## Side Effects and Drug Interactions

### Salicylates and NSAIDs

The most common side effect of the salicylates and the NSAIDs is stomach upset. Therefore you should take these medications with food. If you have an ulcer condition, your doctor may want you to avoid these two categories of pain relievers altogether. The important thing is to check with your doctor before you take a nonprescription drug product that contains aspirin or ibuprofen. Of the three nonprescription pain relievers on the market, acetaminophen is the one that is least likely to aggravate ulcers.

Nonprescription muscle-ache liniments that are applied to the skin, such as Ben-Gay or Icy-Hot, contain salicylates that can be absorbed into the bloodstream if you overuse them. If you combine these linaments with high doses of aspirin, you may experience such side effects as ringing in the ears and dizziness.

## Narcotic Pain Relievers and Muscle Relaxants

The most common side effects of the narcotic pain relievers and the muscle relaxants are drowsiness and dizziness. Therefore, use caution if you have to drive your car or do other tasks that require mental alertness.

Check with your doctor before taking other drug products that may cause drowsiness. Combining two medications that each cause drowsiness may make you feel oversedated and very dizzy.

If you are taking a narcotic pain reliever, such as codeine, over several days or weeks, you may become constipated. In that case you may want to take a stool softener (such as Colace) or increase your intake of dietary fiber. Ask your pharmacist to recommend a stool softener or laxative for you.

## Gout Medications

Anturane and Benemid may be less effective if you take aspirin or other salicylates with them. Therefore, if you are treating a fever, take acetaminophen, which is less likely to interfere with these drugs.

Benemid interacts with other medications by preventing their elimination from the body. A fact of interest, although totally unrelated to pain relief, is that Benemid may be combined with another medication, such as penicillin, to provide high blood levels of that medication—a beneficial drug interaction.

A strange interaction may occur with Zyloprim and ampicillin, an antibiotic—you may develop a skin rash. Why this happens is not clear, but it is thought that people who are sensitive to ampicillin may have a more definite reaction when it is combined with Zyloprim. This is not likely to occur, however, with the other antibiotics in the penicillin family. If you do develop a rash from this combination, contact your doctor right away.

## Rheumatoid Arthritis Drugs

If your Ridaura prescription seems expensive, this should be no surprise—after all, it is literally "made of gold"! Except for one isolated report that gold medications may interact with Dilantin, Ridaura does not appear to interact with other medications.

Methotrexate is also used to treat psoriasis and certain kinds of cancer. See Key 33 for methotrexate drug interactions.

## Ergotamine for Migraine Headache

Ergotamine itself is not a pain reliever, but does help to ease the pain and other symptoms of migraine headache. It acts by constricting blood vessels in the brain that have become overdilated. Interestingly, this is exactly opposite to the way in which nitrates (including nitroglycerin) act to relieve angina pectoris. Combined, ergotamine and nitrates can worsen angina.

### DRUG INTERACTION CHART:
### PAIN RELIEVERS/MUSCLE RELAXANTS/
### MIGRAINE HEADACHE PRODUCTS

| Drug Interaction | Rating* | Potential Effects/Recommendations |
|---|---|---|
| Anturane/Coumadin | A | See Key 19. |
| Anturane/Orinase | A | See Key 28. |
| Anturane/Pepto-Bismol | A | Anturane may be less effective. Ask your pharmacist to help you select an diarrhea medication that does not interact with Anturane. |
| Anturane/Salicylates (Including Aspirin) | A | Anturane may be less effective. If you need a nonprescription pain reliever, ask your pharmacist to help you select a product that does not contain salicylates or aspirin. |

103

| Drug Interaction | Rating* | Potential Effects/Recommendations |
|---|---|---|
| Benemid/Diabinese | D | See Key 28. |
| Benemid/Lufyllin | B | See Key 20. |
| Benemid/Methotrexate | A | See Key 33. |
| Benemid/Penicillin | C | See Key 31. |
| Benemid/Salicylates (Including Aspirin) | A | Benemid may be less effective if taken with high doses of salicylates or aspirin. (Infrequent or low doses of salicyaltes or aspirin are less likely to interfere with your Benemid therapy.) Ask your doctor what dosage of aspirin you may take with Benemid. |
| Butazolidin/Anticoagulants | A | See Key 19. |
| Butazolidin/Barbiturates | D | Butazolidin may be less effective. Contact your doctor if your pain worsens. |
| Butazolidin/Diabetes Medicines | A | See Key 28. |
| Butazolidin/Dilantin | A | See Key 30. |
| Butazolidin/Methotrexate | A | See Key 33. |
| Darvon or Darvocet-N/Barbiturates | C | See Key 22. |
| Demerol/Dilantin | C | Demerol may be less effective. If your pain does not improve, contact your doctor. |
| Demerol/MAOIs | A | See Key 23. |
| Demerol/Thorazine | A | See Key 24. |
| Indocin/Apresoline | B | See Key 12. |
| Indocin/Dyrenium | B | See Key 13. |
| Indocin/Lithium | C | See Key 24. |
| Methadone/Dilantin | A | Methadone may be less effective. If your pain does not improve or you experience other symptoms, contact your doctor. |

| Drug Interaction | Rating* | Potential Effects/Recommendations |
|---|---|---|
| Migraine Headache Medications That Contain Ergotamine/ Erythromycin | A | Ergotamine may have a more potent effect. If your hands or feet feel numb or cold or turn blue, contact your doctor *right away*. |
| Migraine Headache Medications That Contain Ergotamine/ Inderal | B | See Key 14. |
| Migraine Headache Medications That Contain Ergotamine/ Nitroglycerin | A | See Key 15. |
| Muscle Relaxants/ Antihistamines | A | Drowsiness and lack of coordination may occur when these medications are taken together. Check with your doctor before taking a nonprescription antihistamine with your muscle relaxant. |
| Naprosyn (Anaprox)/ Benemid | C | Naprosyn may have a more potent effect. Your doctor may adjust your Naprosyn dosage when you start or stop taking Benemid. |
| Narcotic Pain Relievers/Alcohol | A | You may become excessively drowsy or dizzy and lose your sense of coordination. Ask your doctor whether you may drink alcoholic beverages with your pain medication and, if so, what quantity is safe. |
| Narcotic Pain Relievers/Reglan | D | You may experience increased sedation, dizziness, and loss of coordination. The dosage of the pain reliever may have to be adjusted. |
| Narcotic Pain Relievers/Tagamet | B | You may experience increased sedation, dizziness, and loss of coordination. The dosage of the pain reliever may have to be adjusted. |
| NSAIDs/ACE Inhibitors | A | See Key 12. |
| NSAIDs/Anticoagulants | C | See Key 19. |

105

| Drug Interaction | Rating* | Potential Effects/Recommendations |
|---|---|---|
| NSAIDs/Beta Blockers | C | See Key 14. |
| NSAIDs/Bumex | C | See Key 13. |
| NSAIDs/Corticosteroids | C | You may experience stomach upset. Take both medications on a full stomach, right after a meal. If you feel intestinal pain, contact your doctor. |
| NSAIDs/Lasix | C | See Key 13. |
| NSAIDs/Methotrexate | A | See Key 33. |
| NSAIDs/Minipress | D | See Key 12. |
| Norflex/Darvon or Darvocet-N | D | Although this drug interaction rarely occurs, you may feel anxious or confused or experience tremors. If you experience any of these side effects, contact your doctor. |
| Norflex/Phenothiazines | C | See Key 24. |
| Norflex/Symmetrel | D | You may experience dry mouth, blurred vision, drowsiness, and dizziness. If you do, contact your doctor. Your Norflex dosage may have to be adjusted. |
| Orudis/Benemid | C | Orudis may have a more potent effect. Your doctor may adjust the dosage of Orudis when you start or stop Benemid. |
| Salicylates/Antacids | D | If you are taking large dosages of a salicylate, the pain killer may be less effective. If your pain worsens, tell your doctor that you are taking both medications. Your doctor may adjust the salicylate dosage. |
| Salicylates/ Corticosteroids | A | If you are taking large dosages of a salicylate and start taking a steroid, the salicylate may be less effective. Once your doctor adjusts your salicylate dosage, *do not* stop taking the steroid medication without your doctor's permission. Doing so can lead to salicylate side effects. |

| Drug Interaction | Rating* | Potential Effects/Recommendations |
|---|---|---|
| Salicylates/Diabetes Medicines | A | See Key 28. |
| Zyloprim/ACE Inhibitors | B | See Key 12. |
| Zyloprim/Ampicillin | C | If you develop a skin rash while taking these medications together, contact your doctor. |
| Zyloprim/Antacids | C | Zyloprim may be less effective if taken with antacids that contain aluminum. To minimize this interaction, take Zyloprim at least three hours before the antacid. |
| Zyloprim/ Anticoagulants | D | See Key 19. |
| Zyloprim/Cytoxan | D | See Key 33. |
| Zyloprim/Diabinese | D | See Key 28. |
| Zyloprim/Dilantin | D | See Key 30. |
| Zyloprim/Imuran | A | See Key 34. |
| Zyloprim/Thiazides | B | See Key 13. |

* The rating indicates how harmful a drug interaction may be and how frequently it may occur.

"A" indicates a drug interaction that may cause serious harm and occurs frequently. "B" indicates a drug interaction that may cause serious harm but occurs less frequently. "C" indicates a drug interaction that is less harmful but occurs frequently. "D" indicates a drug interaction that is less harmful and occurs less frequently. See Key 9 for more information about the rating system.

# 27

# PRESCRIPTION COUGH/COLD/ ALLERGY MEDICATIONS

Red, itchy, watery eyes, postnasal drip, nasal congestion, sneezing, and coughing are symptoms familiar to everyone. Sometimes, it's hard to tell if they are due to an *allergy* or a *cold*. What's the difference? The difference may be in the drug treatment.

An allergy is caused by the body's reaction to an "allergen"—a foreign substance, such as pollen, that has entered your body. In response to the allergen, your body triggers a sequence of reactions that, in the end, causes the release of *histamine*. Histamine, a substance found in all body tissues, is responsible for among other things, dilating blood vessels in the nose. This dilation is what causes the nasal congestion we're all familiar with. The best treatment for most allergies, as you may have guessed, is an *anti*histamine! Decongestants are often added to allergy drug products to relieve nasal stuffiness. Allergies may be seasonal or may last all year round.

Colds are caused by viruses and usually last about 7 to 14 days. Unlike the situation with bacterial infections, no medications that can *cure* a cold are available. (There are medications that may minimize the severity of the symptoms of a cold, but they will not cure the cold once you've got it.) Most cold products contain a cough suppressant (to stop excessive coughing), an expectorant (to thin bronchial congestion), and a decongestant. Some also contain an antihistamine.

Unfortunately, there's nothing you can do to defeat a cold except rest, drink fluids, and treat the symptoms—with a cough medicine, vaporizer, and chicken soup—which will at least make you feel better!

108

# The Medications

Cough, cold, and allergy medications (or ingredients) are as follows:

1. antihistamines: *chlorpheniramine, Clistin, diphenydramine, Hismanal, Optimine, PBZ, Periactin, Phenergan, Polaraime, promethazine, Seldane, Tacaryl, Tavist,* and *Temaril.*
2. decongestants: *phenylephrine, phenylpropranolamine (PPA),* and *pseudoephedrine.*
3. cough suppressants: *codeine, dextromethorphan,* and *Tessalon Perles.*
4. expectorants: *guaifenesin, Organidin,* and *SSKI.*

Most prescription drug products contain more than one ingredient. Here are some examples:

*Ambenyl* = codeine + bromodiphenhyramine (antihistamine)

*Bromphed* = pseudoephedrine + brompheniramine (antihistmine)

*Comhist LA* = phenylephrine + chlorpheniriamine + phenyltoloxamine (antihistamine)

*Entex LA* = PPA + guaifenesin

*Naldecon* = PPA + phenylephrine + chlorpheniramine + phenyltoloxamine

*Nolamine* = PPA + chlorpheniramine + phenindamine (antihistmine)

*Novahistine DH* = pseudoephedrine + chlorpheniramine + codeine

*Phenergan VC with Codeine* = phenylephrine + Phenergan + codeine

*Rynatan* = phenylephrine + chlorpheniramine + pyrilamine (antihistamine)

*Tavist D* = PPA + Tavist

*Tussi-Organidin* = Organidin + codeine

*Tussi-Organidin DM* = Organidin + dextromethorphan

*Tuss-Ornade Spansules* = PPA + caramiphen (cough suppressent)

## Side Effects and Drug Interactions

### Antihistamines

The most common side effects of the antihistamines, except Seldane and Hismanal, are drowsiness and dizziness. Reaction time may also be reduced or delayed, especially in persons who are age 50 or older. Therefore, it is important to use caution if you have to drive your car.

Combining antihistamines with other medications that also cause drowsiness may lead to extreme sedation, weakness, and loss of coordination. Also, many nonprescription drug products contain antihistamines, so check with your doctor or pharmacist before you combine your prescribed medication with other drug products.

Seldane and Hismanal are two antihistamines that usually do not cause drowiness. Drug interactions for Hismanal have not yet been reported, although Hismanal has been shown to interact with food. Approximately 60 percent of the drug may be destroyed by food before it has a chance to be absorbed into the bloodstream, and this may reduce its effectiveness.

Seldane has been shown to interact with Nizoral, a fungal medication; the combination may cause heart abnormalities.

### Decongestants

The most common side effects of decongestants are nervousness and insomnia. If you are having trouble sleeping, do not take a decongestant at night. Decongestants may interact with blood pressure medications, causing increased blood pressure. Therefore, if you are taking a blood pressure medication, do not take a decongestant without first checking with your doctor.

Many nonprescription diet aids also contain phenylpropranolamine (PPA), so check the active ingredients (or ask your pharmacist to help you) before you combine your cough/cold/allergy medication with a diet aid.

## Cough Suppressants

The most common side effects of codeine are drowsiness, dizziness, and constipation.

Tessalon Perles come in capsule form. Be sure not to chew the capsule—it is very bitter.

## Expectorants

Expectorants that contain iodides, such as Organidin and SSKI, may affect your thyroid if they are overused. Be sure to follow the dosage that your doctor has ordered. Drink plenty of water throughout the day; water helps the expectorant to break up bronchial mucus.

### DRUG INTERACTION CHART:
### PRESCRIPTION COUGH/COLD/
### ALLERGY MEDICATIONS

| Drug Interaction | Rating* | Potential Effects/Recommendations |
| --- | --- | --- |
| Antihistamines/ Antispasmodics | C | See Key 11. |
| Antihistamines/ Compazine | A | See Key 24 and Key 25, "Phenothiazines/Antihistamines." |
| Antihistamines/ Phenothiazines | A | See Key 24. |
| Antihistamines/ Reglan | D | See Key 11. |
| Antihistamines/ Sleep Aids | A | See Key 38. |
| Antihistamines/ Thorazine | A | See Key 24 and Key 25, "Phenothiazines/ Antihistamines." |
| Antihistamines/ Transderm Scōp | A | See Key 25. |
| Decongestants/ Aldomet | A | See Key 12. |
| Decongestants/ Beta Blockers | B | See Key 14. |
| Decongestants/ Ismelin | C | See Key 12. |
| Decongestants/MAOIs | A | See Key 23. |

| Drug Interaction | Rating* | Potential Effects/Recommendations |
|---|---|---|
| Decongestants/ Reserpine | B | See Key 12. |
| Decongestants/TCAs | A | See Key 23. |
| Hismanal/Food | A | Hismanal may not be absorbed and may therefore be less effective. Take Hismanal one to two hours before your meal. |
| Organidin/Lithium | B | If you are susceptible to hypothyroidism, this combination could affect your iodine balance. If you have a thyroid condition, be sure to tell your doctor. |
| Phenergan/Lithium | B | You may feel disoriented or may experience involuntary muscle movements. If these symptoms occur, contact your doctor *immediately*. |
| Seldane/Nizoral | A | The combination of these two medications may lead to heart abnormalities. Do not take Seldane with Nizoral unless your doctor tells you to do so. |
| Tussi-Organidin or Tussi-Organidin DM/ Lithium | B | If you are susceptible to hypothyroidism, this combination could affect your iodine balance. If you have a thyroid condition, be sure to tell your doctor. |

* The rating indicates how harmful a drug interaction may be and how frequently it may occur.

"A" indicates a drug interaction that may cause serious harm and occurs frequently. "B" indicates a drug interaction that may cause serious harm but occurs less frequently. "C" indicates a drug interaction that is less harmful but occurs frequently. "D" indicates a drug interaction that is less harmful and occurs less frequently. See Key 9 for more information about the rating system.

# INSULIN AND OTHER MEDICATIONS FOR DIABETES

*Diabetes mellitus* (commonly referred to as "diabetes") is a disorder in which the body lacks insulin, a hormone needed to change sugars and carbohydrates into a form that the body can store for use at another time.

Insulin is normally secreted from the pancreas and then interacts with sugars and carbohydrates to change them. However, in people who have diabetes, either enough insulin may not be secreted, or it may not be able to interact with sugars and carbohydrates. In either case, the blood becomes overloaded with sugars, which then spill into the urine.

Symptoms of diabetes include increased urination, increased thirst and hunger, weight loss, sugar in the urine, and high blood sugar level (an abnormally high amount of sugar in the bloodstream). Treatment may involve an oral diabetes medication or insulin.

Glucagon, another hormone naturally secreted by the pancreas, plays a role opposite to that of insulin: it takes sugars and carbohydrates out of storage so that the body can use them for energy. Glucagon is available in injectable form. It is reserved for emergency use when the blood sugar level dips too low, resulting in a *hypoglycemic reaction* (weakness, sweating, headache, increased heart rate, confusion, dizziness, loss of consciousness). Glucose tablets are also available for this purpose but cannot be given to people who are unconscious.

## The Medications

There are three categories of diabetes medicines:

1. oral diabetes medicines: *chlorpropamide, Diabeta, Diabinese, Dymelor, Glucotrol, Micronase, Orinase, tolbutamide,* and *Tolinase.*

2. *insulin.*
3. *glucagon.*
4. *glucose: Glutose, Insta-Glucose,* and *Insulin Reaction* liquids, and *B-D Glucose* chewable tablets.

## Side Effects and Drug Interactions

Treating diabetes is like performing a balancing act. The diabetic patient must take the right dosage of medication to offset the amount of sugar or other food eaten. Exercise and other medications that interact with diabetes medications are also important factors. Unbalanced, the scale can tip either way, resulting in hypoglycemia or hyperglycemia.

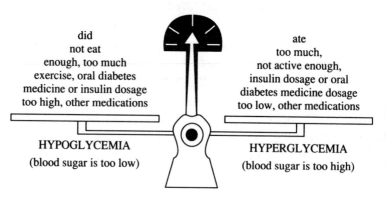

did not eat enough, too much exercise, oral diabetes medicine or insulin dosage too high, other medications

ate too much, not active enough, insulin dosage or oral diabetes medicine dosage too low, other medications

HYPOGLYCEMIA
(blood sugar is too low)

HYPERGLYCEMIA
(blood sugar is too high)

If you are being treated for diabetes, you are probably already checking your blood sugar level or the amount of sugar in your urine on a regular basis. It is especially important to check for a change in your glucose level when you add a new medication to your drug treatment, or when you stop taking a drug that was part of your regimen.

If you check the drug interaction chart, you may be surprised to see how many medications can change the potency of your insulin or diabetes medicine. Your doctor may have to adjust the dosage of one or more of your medications whenever a change in medication is made. To avoid losing of control of your blood sugar, be sure to take all of your medications exactly as your doctor has prescribed, and do not skip doses.

114

# DRUG INTERACTION CHART:
## INSULIN AND OTHER MEDICATIONS FOR DIABETES

| Drug Interaction | Rating* | Potential Effects/Recommendations |
| --- | --- | --- |
| Diabetes Medicines/ Alcohol | A | Excessive amounts of alcohol can lead to hypoglycemia (low blood sugar) in those who are taking Glucatrol. People who are taking Orinase may experience increased blood sugar if they drink excessive amounts of alcohol. Those who are taking Diabinese may experience headache and flushing of the face. Ask your doctor whether you may drink alcoholic beverages with your medication and, if so, what quantity is safe. |
| Diabetes Medicines/ Aldomet | D | The diabetes medication may have a more potent effect, which can lead to hypoglycemia (low blood sugar). Check your blood sugar when you start or stop Aldomet. |
| Diabetes Medicines/ Aspirin | A | The diabetes medication, especially Diabinese, may have a more potent effect when combined with large amounts of aspirin. Ask your doctor whether you may take aspirin with your diabetes medicine. Beware: some nonprescription drug products contain aspirin! Check the ingredients, or ask your pharmacist to make sure the product you've selected does not contain aspirin. |
| Diabetes Medicines/ Atromid S | D | Diabetes drugs, including insulin, may have a more potent effect. Check blood sugar levels and watch for hypoglycemia (low blood sugar) when Atromid S is started or stopped. |
| Diabetes Medicines/ Butazolidin | A | The diabetes medication may have a more potent effect, which can lead to hypoglycemia (low blood sugar). Your doctor may want to check your blood |

| Drug Interaction | Rating* | Potential Effects/Recommendations |
|---|---|---|
| | | sugar level when you start or stop Butazolidin, and may adjust the dosage of the diabetes drug. |
| Diabetes Medicines/ Capoten | D | Diabetes medications, including insulin, may have a more potent effect. Your doctor may want to check your blood sugar level when you start Capoten. |
| Diabetes Medicines/ Catapres | D | Although Catapres will not alter the effects of diabetes medications, it may conceal the symptoms of hypoglycemia (low blood sugar). Consequently, if your blood sugar drops too low, you may not have symptoms of sweating or fast heart rate to warn you. |
| Diabetes Medicines/ Charcoal | A | The diabetes medication may not be fully absorbed and may therefore be less effective. Ask your pharmacist to help you select an intestinal gas medication that does not contain charcoal. |
| Diabetes Medicines/ Corticosteroids | C | The diabetes medication may be less effective, and your blood sugar level may increase. Your doctor may want to check your blood sugar level when you start, stop, or change the dosage of the corticosteroid. |
| Diabetes Medicines/ Digoxin | D | See Key 17. |
| Diabetes Medicines/ Ismelin | D | The diabetes medication may have a more potent effect. Check your blood sugar level when you start or stop Ismelin. |
| Diabetes Medicines/ Potassium Supplements | D | If your potassium blood level is low, and you are being treated with potassium supplements, your blood sugar may drop. Check your blood sugar regularly. |
| Diabetes Medicines/ Rifampin | C | Diabeta, Diabinese, Orinase and Micronase may be less effective, which can lead to increased blood sugar |

| Drug Interaction | Rating* | Potential Effects/Recommendations |
|---|---|---|
| | | levels. Your doctor may want to check your blood sugar level when you start or stop Rifampin, and may adjust the dosage of your diabetes medication. |
| Diabetes Medicines/ Salicylates | A | The diabetes medication, especially Diabinese, may have a more potent effect when combined with large amounts of salicylates. Many nonprescription drug products, including arthritis/muscle ache creams, contain salicylates. Be sure to ask your doctor whether you can use these products with your diabetes medication. |
| Diabetes Medicines/ Sulfonamides | C | The diabetes medication may have a more potent effect which can lead to hypoglycemia (low blood sugar). Check your blood sugar while you are taking a sulfonamide antibiotic. (Diabeta and Micronase do not interact). |
| Diabetes Medicines/ Tagamet | D | The diabetes medication may have a more potent effect, which can lead to hypoglycemia (low blood sugar). Check your blood sugar level regularly. |
| Diabetes Medicines/ TCAs | D | Diabetes medications, inlucing insulin, may have a more potent effect. Check your blood sugar level when you start, stop, or change the dosage of the antidepressant. |
| Diabetes Medicines/ Thiazides | C | Your blood sugar may increase. Your doctor may want to check your blood sugar regularly and may adjust the dosage of your diabetes medication. |
| Diabetes Medicines/ Thorazine | D | Large doses of Thorazine may cause your blood sugar level to increase. Your doctor may check your blood sugar level regularly. |

117

| Drug Interaction | Rating* | Potential Effects/Recommendations |
|---|---|---|
| Diabetes Medicines/ Thyroid Replacement Medications | D | The diabetes medication may be less effective when you start taking thyroid replacement drugs such as Synthroid, thyroid, or Thyrolar. Your doctor may want to check your blood sugar when you start or change the dosage of thyroid medications. |
| Diabinese/Benemid | D | Diabinese may have a more potent effect which can lead to hypoglycemia (low blood sugar). Check your blood sugar level when you start Benemid. |
| Diabinese/Zyloprim | D | Diabinese may have a more potent effect which can lead to hypoglycemia (low blood sugar). Check your blood sugar level when you start Zyloprim. |
| Glucagon/Coumadin | B | See Key 19. |
| Insulin/Alcohol | A | Insulin may have a more potent effect if you ingest alcohol on an empty stomach. With your doctor's permission, drink no more than moderate amounts of alcohol and only with meals. |
| Insulin/Beta Blockers (Nonselective) | A | If your blood sugar is too low, you may not experience some of the characteristic symptoms of hypoglycemia (low blood sugar). Sweating usually does occur; however, tachycardia (fast heartbeat) may not. Check your blood sugar regularly. |
| Insulin/Ismelin | B | Your blood sugar may decrease when you start Ismelin or increase when you stop Ismelin. Check your blood sugar regularly. |

| Drug Interaction | Rating* | Potential Effects/Recommendations |
|---|---|---|
| Insulin/Smoking | A | If you are a heavy smoker, you may require more insulin. Therefore, if you change your smoking habits, your insulin requirements may change. If you plan to quit smoking, do it under the supervision of your doctor—good luck! |
| Insulin/ The Tetracyclines | D | Insulin may have a more potent effect which may lead to hypoglycemia (low blood sugar). Check your blood sugar level regularly. |
| Orinase/Anturane | A | Orinase may have a more potent effect which may lead to hypoglycemia (low blood sugar). Check your blood sugar level regularly. |

* The rating indicates how harmful a drug interaction may be and how frequently it may occur.

"A" indicates a drug interaction that may cause serious harm and occurs frequently. "B" indicates a drug interaction that may cause serious harm but occurs less frequently. "C" indicates a drug interaction that is less harmful but occurs frequently. "D" indicates a drug interaction that is less harmful and occurs less frequently. See Key 9 for more information about the rating system.

# 29

# CORTICOSTEROIDS/THYROID MEDICATIONS/ESTROGENS

The *corticosteroids* are used in the treatment of many different kinds of diseases and ailments—asthma, arthritis, ulcerative colitis, allergic reactions, poison ivy, and skin rashes, to name just a few. Corticosteroids relieve these conditions by reducing inflammation and swelling. If you have ever used a Medrol Dosepak to get rid of poison ivy, you've probably seen first hand how effective corticosteroids can be!

*Thyroid hormone* is necessary for growth and metabolism in the body. It is secreted by the thyroid gland and contains iodine. Three thyroid disorders are *hypothyroidism* (not enough thyroid secreted), *hyperthyroidism* (too much thyroid secreted), and *thyroiditis* (swelling and pain of the thyroid gland). *Grave's disease*, shared by President George Bush and his wife, Barbara, is another, and is caused by excessive thyroid secretion.

The *estrogens* may be prescribed for postmenopausal women for the following purposes:

1. to relieve "hot flashes" after menopause.
2. to serve as a replacement hormone to prevent bone loss in women who are susceptible to osteoporosis.
3. to treat atrophic vaginitis, a condition in which the walls of the vagina lose elasticity and become inflamed.
4. to treat breast cancer.

Estrogens are also used for prostate cancer in men. (Birth control pills are not included in this Key because they are beyond the scope of this book.)

## The Medications

1. The corticosteroids include *Aristocort, Celestone, Cortef, cortisone, Decadron, Deltasone, dexamethasone,*

*Hexadrol, hydrocortisone, Medrol, methylpredniso-lone, Orasone, prednisone, prednisolone,* and *triamcinolone.*

2. The thyroid medications include:
   a. thyroid replacement hormones: *Armour Thyroid, Cytomel, Euthroid, levothyroxine, Levoxin, Proloid, Synthroid, thyroid,* and *Thyrolar.*
   b. iodine replacement therapy: *Lugol's Solution,* and *Strong Iodine Solution.*
   c. hyperthyroid medications: *propylthiouricil (PTU),* and *Tapazole.*
3. The estrogens include *conjugated estrogens, Estinyl, Estratab, Ogen,* and *Premarin.*

## Side Effects and Drug Interactions

### Corticosteroids

Corticosteroids seem to have a bad reputation—some people refuse to have their steroid prescriptions filled because they've "heard so many bad things about them." In reality, if these persons would take their medications exactly as their doctors have prescribed, most of them would find relief for their medical problems, with minimal side effects.

The most common side effect of the corticosteroids is stomach upset, which can be minimized by taking the drug with food. A side effect that may occur if the corticosteroid is not taken correctly is a feeling of disorientation. This once happened to a female patient who "did not like taking pills." She received a corticosteroid for her asthma and was instructed by her doctor to take six tablets daily for the first five days, five tablets daily for the next five days, four tablets daily for the next five days, and so on. However, after two weeks, her asthma symptoms lessened, so she decided to stop taking the pills. The next day, she felt disoriented and "not right."

Stopping medication after your symptoms are gone is not unusual—it even makes sense! With corticosteroids, however, it is necessary most of the time to taper off the dosage, or side effects may occur.

## Thyroid Medications

Thyroid medications may change the potency of other medications, such as digoxin and anticoagulants. Therefore, your doctor may want to check on the effectiveness of all of your medications when you start, stop, or change the dosage of your thyroid medication.

## Estrogens

You may have heard that estrogens interact with many other medications. However, those drug interactions involve the birth control pill and may result in reduced effectiveness and increased risk of pregnancy. These drug interactions do not apply to the woman who is taking estrogen as a replacement hormone or as a supplement to prevent osteoporosis.

### DRUG INTERACTION CHART: CORTICOSTEROIDS/THYROID MEDICATIONS/ ESTROGENS

| Drug Interaction | Rating* | Potential Effects/Recommendations |
|---|---|---|
| Corticosteroids/ Anticoagulants | D | See Key 19. |
| Corticosteroids/ Aspirin | A | See Key 35. |
| Corticosteroids/ Barbiturates | C | The corticosteroid may be less effective. Your doctor may adjust the dosage of the corticosteroid if a barbiturate is added to your therapy. |
| Corticosteroids/ Diabetes Medicines | C | See Key 28. |
| Corticosteroids/ Dilantin | A | The corticosteroid may be less effective a few days after you start taking both medications together. Your doctor may adjust the dosage of the corticosteroid. |

| Drug Interaction | Rating* | Potential Effects/Recommendations |
|---|---|---|
| Corticosteroids/ Estrogens | C | The corticosteroid may have a more potent effect. Your doctor may adjust the dosage of the corticosteroid. |
| Corticosteroids/ Mysoline | C | The corticosteroid may be less effective. Your doctor may adjust the corticosteroid dosage when Mysoline is added to your drug treatment. |
| Corticosteroids/ Nizoral | A | Medrol, prednisone, and prednisolone may have more potent effects. Your doctor may adjust the corticosteroid dosage when you start or stop Nizoral. |
| Corticosteroids/NSAIDs | C | See Key 26. |
| Corticosteroids/ Rifampin | A | The corticosteroid may be less effective. Your doctor may adjust the corticosteroid dosage while you are taking rifampin. |
| Corticosteroids/ Salicylates | A | See Key 26. |
| Corticosteroids/ Sandimmune | B | This combination is often prescribed after organ transplants. However, both the corticosteroid and Sandimmune may have more potent effects when they are combined. Your doctor may want to check your drug therapy frequently and may adjust the dosage of one or both drugs. |
| Corticosteroids/ Tegretol | A | The corticosteroid may be less effective. Your doctor may adjust the corticosteroid dosage. Do not skip doses of either medication. |
| Decadron/Antacids | D | Decadron may be less effective. Your doctor may want to see you regularly to check on Decadron's effectiveness. |
| Decacron/Cytadren | A | Decadron may be less effective. Your doctor may adjust your Decadron dosage. |

123

| Drug Interaction | Rating* | Potential Effects/Recommendations |
|---|---|---|
| Estrogens/Atromid S | D | See Key 18. |
| Estrogens/ Benzodiazepines | D | See Key 21. |
| Hydrocortisone/ Questran | B | Hydrocortisone may be less effective. Take hydrocortisone two hours before or after Questran. |
| Medrol/Erythromycin | B | Medrol may have a more potent effect. If you are taking Medrol every day for several weeks, and you start taking erythromycin, your doctor may want to check your Medrol dosage. |
| Propylthiouricil (PTU)/ Anticoagulants | A | See Key 19. |
| Propylthiouricil (PTU)/ Digoxin | A | See Key 17. |
| Propylthiouricil (PTU)/ Theophylline | C | See Key 20. |
| Tapazole/ Anticoagulants | A | See Key 19. |
| Tapazole/Digoxin | A | See Key 17. |
| Thyroid/Anticoagulants | A | See Key 19. |
| Thyroid/Diabetes Medicines | D | See Key 28. |
| Thyroid/Digoxin | A | See Key 17. |
| Thyroid/Mevacor | B | Thyroid may have a more potent action or be less effective when combined with Mevacor. Your doctor may want to check your thyroid dosage frequently when you start taking Mevacor. |
| Thyroid/Questran | A | Thyroid binds with Questran in the intestinal tract, may not be completely absorbed, and may be less effective. Take thyroid six hours before or after Questran. |

| Drug Interaction | Rating* | Potential Effects/Recommendations |
|---|---|---|
| Thyroid/Tegretol | C | Thyroid may be less effective. Your doctor may want to check your thyroid dosage regularly. |
| Thyroid/Theophylline | C | See Key 20. |

\* The rating indicates how harmful a drug interaction may be and how frequently it may occur.

"A" indicates a drug interaction that may cause serious harm and occurs frequently. "B" indicates a drug interaction that may cause serious harm but occurs less frequently. "C" indicates a drug interaction that is less harmful but occurs frequently. "D" indicates a drug interaction that is less harmful and occurs less frequently. See Key 9 for more information about the rating system.

# 30

# ANTICONVULSANTS TO CONTROL EPILEPSY

When you think of the term "seizure," you may envision someone moving violently and uncontrollably back and forth as if he's been electrocuted. This may be a good description of a person who is suffering from a generalized tonic-clonic seizure (formally known as "grand mal"), but there are other types of epilepsy in which different kinds of seizures may take place. For example, some people may suffer from absence seizures (formally known as "petit mal") which may go unnoticed by other people.

*Epilepsy*, in all of its forms, may be described as a disorder in which nerve cells in the brain fire uncontrolled electrical discharges, resulting in loss of consciousness and seizures. Although the occurrence of seizures tends to be unpredictable, some people may experience sensations or visual disturbances, such as an "aura," which may indicate that a seizure is coming on.

## The Medications

The most commonly prescribed anticonvulsants are as follows:

1. *Dilantin.*
2. barbiturates: *Mebaral* and *phenobarbital*, discussed in Key 22.
3. benzodiazepines: *diazepam, Klonopin, Tranxene,* and *Valium,* discussed in Key 21.
4. succinimides: *Celontin* and *Zarontin.*
5. miscellaneous: *carbamazepine, Depakene, Depakote, Mysoline,* and *Tegretol.*

Your drug treatment may include one or more of these medications, depending on the severity and type of seizures you have.

## Side Effects and Drug Interactions

To reduce seizures and minimize any side effects of your seizure medication, your doctor must determine what dosage is correct for you. If the dosage is too high, you may experience side effects caused by the drug; if it is too low, the drug may not be effective in reducing your seizures.

### Dilantin

Finding the correct dosage for Dilantin may be tricky, because side effects can occur very close to the dosage needed to control seizures. In other words, for Dilantin, unlike most medications, there isn't a large difference between the dosage required for treatment and the dosage that produces side effects.

Dosing may become even more difficult when other medications are added to your drug therapy, because they too may change the potency of Dilantin, thereby making it less effective or more potent (with increased chance of side effects).

Because dosing is so critical with Dilantin therapy, your doctor may want to check your Dilantin blood level regularly. In that way, if your blood level measurement is too high or low, your doctor can adjust the dosage.

The most common side effects of Dilantin are as follows:

1. *ataxia* (a lack of coordination that may result in loss of balance or staggered gait).
2. *nystagmus* (an involuntary, rhythmic movement of the eyes).
3. dizziness, slurred speech, nervousness, muscle twitching, and mental confusion.

Contact your doctor *immediately* if you experience any of these side effects, especially if they occur after another medication has been added to your drug therapy.

**Tegretol**

The most common side effects of Tegretol are drowsiness and dizziness. Other side effects, such as nausea, vomiting, confusion, and lack of coordination, may also occur, especially if Tegretol becomes more potent as the result of a drug interaction with another medication.

**Anticonvulsants in general**

As you look down the drug interaction chart, you may notice that some *anticonvulsant* drugs (those used for seizures) interact with other anticonvulsants. For example, Dilantin and Mysoline interact to produce a more potent effect of each drug—an example of a beneficial drug interaction. Such combinations of drugs are often prescribed.

There is one dangerous side effect not yet mentioned that can occur with your anticonvulsant therapy: if you stop taking your anticonvulsant abruptly, you may be more likely to have a seizure or a series of seizures. Because epilepsy is a serious disorder, and the anticonvultant dosages are so critical, it is important that you take your medication *exactly as your doctor has instructed*. Be sure not to skip doses and follow through with appointments to have your drug blood level checked regularly if necessary.

## DRUG INTERACTION CHART:
## ANTICONVULSANTS TO CONTROL EPILEPSY

| Drug Interaction | Rating* | Potential Effects/Recommendations |
| --- | --- | --- |
| Depakene/Antacids | D | Depakene may have a more potent effect. Take Depakene one hour before or two hours after the antacid to minimize the effects of this drug interaction. |
| Depakene/Aspirin | A | Depakene may have a more potent effect. Ask your doctor whether you may take aspirin with Depakene and, if so, what dosage. Many pain relievers and cold/allergy products contain aspirin or aspirinlike ingredients. Ask your pharmacist to help you select a pain reliever or cold product that will not interact. |

| Drug Interaction | Rating* | Potential Effects/Recommendations |
| --- | --- | --- |
| Depakene/Charcoal | A | Depakene may not be completely absorbed and may therefore be less effective. Ask your pharmacist to help you select an intestinal gas medication that does not contain charcoal. |
| Depakene/Mysoline | A | See Key 22. |
| Depakene/Phenobarbital | A | See Key 22. |
| Depakene/Tagamet | D | Depakene may have a more potent effect. Your doctor may want to examine you and check your Depakene blood levels regularly, especially if you are being treated with a high dosage of the anticonvulsant. |
| Depakene/Tegretol | C | Depakene may be less effective. Your doctor may want to examine you and check your blood levels regularly after you start taking the medications together. |
| Depakene/Thorazine | C | Depakene may have a more potent effect. Your doctor may adjust your dosage. |
| Dilantin/Alcohol | C | Dilantin may be less effective if you drink large amounts of alcohol. Ask your doctor whether you may drink alcoholic beverages with Dilantin, and if so, what quantity is safe. |
| Dilantin/Antacids | D | Dilantin may not be completely absorbed and may be less effective. Take the antacid several hours before or after Dilantin. |
| Dilantin/Anticoagulants | B | Dilantin may have a more potent effect; the effectiveness of the anticoagulant may also change. Your doctor may want to check your Dilantin blood level and your prothrombin time regularly. |

| Drug Interaction | Rating* | Potential Effects/Recommendations |
|---|---|---|
| Dilantin/Butazolidin | A | Dilantin may have a more potent effect. Your doctor may want to check your Dilantin blood level and may adjust the dosage. Contact your doctor if you experience Dilantin side effects. |
| Dilantin/Carafate | C | Dilantin may be less effective. Take Dilantin two hours before or after Carafate to minimize this interaction. |
| Dilantin/Celontin | C | Dilantin may have a more potent effect. Your doctor may adjust your Dilantin dosage. |
| Dilantin/Charcoal | A | Dilantin may not be completely absorbed and may therefore be less effective. Ask your pharmacist to help you select an intestinal gas medication that does not contain charcoal. |
| Dilantin/Chlor-Trimeton | D | Dilantin may have a more potent effect. Ask your pharmacist to help you select a nonprescription cold/allergy product that does not contain chlorpheniramine, the antihistamine in Chlor-Trimeton allergy/cold products. |
| Dilantin/Corticosteroids | A | See Key 29. |
| Dilantin/Demerol | C | See Key 26. |
| Dilantin/Depakene | A | Dilantin may have a more potent effect, and Depakene may be less effective. Your doctor may want to check the blood levels of both medications regularly and may adjust the dosage of each. |
| Dilantin/Diflucan | A | Dilantin may have a more potent effect. Your doctor may check your Dilantin blood level regularly and adjust your dosage. Contact your doctor if you experience Dilantin side effects such as dizziness, confusion, and slurred speech. |
| Dilantin/Digoxin | D | See Key 17. |

| Drug Interaction | Rating* | Potential Effects/Recommendations |
|---|---|---|
| Dilantin/Flagyl | D | Dilantin may have a more potent effect. If you are taking high dosages of Dilantin, your doctor may want to check your Dilantin blood levels and may adjust the dosage. |
| Dilantin/Folic Acid | B | Dilantin may be less effective when combined with high dosages of folic acid. |
| Dilantin/Haldol | D | See Key 24. |
| Dilantin/Ibuprofen | D | Dilantin may have a more potent effect when combined with large doses of ibuprofen. Ask your doctor whether you may take ibuprofen with Dilantin and, if so, what dosage is correct. |
| Dilantin/Isoniazid (INH) | A | Dilantin may have a more potent effect. Your doctor may examine you frequently and may adjust your Dilantin dosage. It is especially important to take each dose of your medication; skipping doses can lead to medication side effects or increased risk of seizures. |
| Dilantin/Levodopa | A | See Key 34. |
| Dilantin/Loxitane | D | Dilantin may be less effective. Your doctor may adjust your Dilantin dosage. |
| Dilantin/Macrodantin | D | Dilantin may be less effective. Your doctor may check your Dilantin blood level when you start or stop Macrodantin. |
| Dilantin/Methadone | A | See Key 26. |
| Dilantin/Methotrexate | A | Dilantin may be less effective. Your doctor may want to check your Dilantin blood level and examine you regularly. The Dilantin dosage may have to be adjusted. |
| Dilantin/Mexitil | A | See Key 16. |
| Dilantin/Mysoline | C | See Key 22. |

131

| Drug Interaction | Rating* | Potential Effects/Recommendations |
|---|---|---|
| Dilantin/Norpace | C | Dilantin may be less effective. You may experience dry mouth, blurred vision, dizziness, and drowsiness caused by Norpace's breakdown product. Contact your doctor if you get these symptoms. |
| Dilantin/Phenothiazines | D | Dilantin may have a more potent effect when combined with Compazine, Mellaril, or Thorazine. The phenothiazine may be less effective. Your doctor may want to examine you regularly. Do not skip doses of either medication. |
| Dilantin/Prilosec | B | Dilantin may have a more potent effect. Your doctor may check your Dilantin blood level and adjust the dosage. |
| Dilantin/Quinidine | A | See Key 16. |
| Dilantin/Rifampin | A | Dilantin may be less effective. Your doctor may want to check your Dilantin blood level and may adjust the dosage. |
| Dilantin/Sandimmune | A | See Key 34. |
| Dilantin/ Sulfonamides | A | Dilantin may have a more potent effect. Your doctor may check your Dilantin blood level and adjust your dosage while you are taking both drugs together. |
| Dilantin/Tagamet | A | Dilantin may have a more potent effect. Your doctor may want to check your Dilantin blood level and may adjust the dosage. Contact your doctor if you experience Dilantin side effects (loss of coordination, confusion). |
| Dilantin/Theophylline | C | See Key 20. |
| Dilantin/Vibramycin | A | See Key 31. |
| Dilantin/Vitamin $B_6$ | C | Dilantin may be less effective when combined with large doses of vitamin $B_6$ over a several-week period. |

| Drug Interaction | Rating* | Potential Effects/Recommendations |
|---|---|---|
| Dilantin/Zarontin | C | Dilantin may have a more potent effect. Your doctor may adjust your Dilantin dosage. |
| Dilantin/Zyloprim | D | Dilantin may have a more potent effect. Your doctor may want to examine you when you start or stop Zyloprim. |
| Tegretol/Anticoagulants | D | See Key 19. |
| Tegretol/CCBs | A | Tegretol may have a more potent effect when combined with Calan (Isoptin) or Cardizem. Your doctor may want to check your Tegretol blood level regularly and may adjust your dosage. (Procardia does not interact with Tegretol.) |
| Tegretol/Charcoal | A | Tegretol may not be completely absorbed and may therefore be less effective. Ask your pharmacist to help you select an intestinal gas medication that does not contain charcoal. |
| Tegretol/ Corticosteroids | A | See Key 29. |
| Tegretol/Darvon or Darvocet-N | A | Tegretol may have a more potent effect, which may lead to Tegretol side effects. If you are seeking medical treatment for a painful condition, be sure your doctor knows that you are taking Tegretol. Do not take pain medications prescribed for other family members or friends. |
| Tegretol/Erythromycin | A | Tegretol may have a more potent effect. Your doctor may check your Tegretol blood level frequently while you are taking erythromycin. If you experience Tegretol side effects, contact your doctor *immediately*. |
| Tegretol/Haldol | C | See Key 24. |

133

| Drug Interaction | Rating* | Potential Effects/Recommendations |
|---|---|---|
| Tegretol/Isoniazid (INH) | A | Both Tegretol and INH may have more potent effects. Your doctor may want to examine you regularly, especially when you start, stop, or change the INH dosage. Do not skip doses of either medication. |
| Tegretol/Lithium | B | See Key 24. |
| Tegretol/Mysoline | C | Tegretol may have a more potent effect; Mysoline may be less effective. Your doctor may want to see you regularly to check the effectiveness of both drugs. |
| Tegretol/Norpramin | D | Tegretol may have a more potent effect. Your doctor may want to examine you regularly. |
| Tegretol/Phenobarbital | C | Tegretol may be less effective. Your doctor may adjust the Tegretol dosage. |
| Tegretol/Phenobarbital | D | See Key 34. |
| Tegretol/Tagamet | A | Tegretol may have a more potent effect if you are already taking this medication and Tagamet is added to your drug therapy. However, Tegretol's increased effect (if it occurs) is usually temporary, and tends to disappear after the first few weeks of treatment. Contact your doctor if you experience Tegretol side effects. |
| Tegretol/Theophylline | D | See Key 20. |
| Tegretol/Thyroid | C | See Key 29. |
| Valium/Digoxin | B | See Key 17, "Digoxin/Valium or Xanax." |

* The rating indicates how harmful a drug interaction may be and how frequently it may occur.

"A" indicates a drug interaction that may cause serious harm and occurs frequently. "B" indicates a drug interaction that may cause serious harm but occurs less frequently. "C" indicates a drug interaction that is less harmful but occurs frequently. "D" indicates a drug interaction that is less harmful and occurs less frequently. See Key 9 for more information about the rating system.

# 31

# ANTIBIOTICS TO TREAT
# INFECTIONS

*Antibiotics* are probably the most frequently prescribed medications—and the variety of antibiotics on the market is astounding! Why do we need so many different kinds? Here's the answer—the bacteria that cause a particular bothersome or life-threatening infection mutate and, in doing so, learn how to live with the antibiotic we are using to cure that infection. In simpler terms, the bacteria become *resistant* to the drug.

Bacterial resistance is a big problem. Most often, it happens when an antibiotic is used many times (sometimes overused). But bacterial resistance may occur simply because the "bugs" are just plain resourceful. You may have seen an example of bacterial resistance first hand if you have a grandchild who gets recurring ear infections. Your grandchild may have received amoxillin for the ear infection. If amoxicillin did not work, the doctor may have prescribed another antibiotic to which the bacteria have not become resistant—yet!

The biggest problem with antibiotics and resistance is that people take antibiotics when it is not appropriate to do so. For example, antibiotics can cure only infections that are caused by bacteria; they are ineffective against viral infections. Nevertheless, many people insist on taking antibiotics (leftover from a previous infection) to "cure" their colds. This is a bad idea for two reasons. First, colds are caused by viruses, and therefore antibiotics will not be effective. Second, as a rule, it is not wise to use medication left over from another illness because it has probably lost its effectiveness.

## The Medications

The most commonly prescribed oral antibiotics are:

1. penicillins: *amoxicillin, ampicillin, Amoxil, Bactocil, Dycill, Dynapen, Nafcil, Omnipen, penicillin, Pen Vee K, Polycillin, Polymox, Tegopen, UniPen,* and *V-Cillin K.*

2. cephalosporins: *Ceclor, cephalexin, Duricef, Keflex, Keftab, Suprax,* and *Velosef.*

3. erythromycin: *E.E.S., E-Mycin, Eyrc, Ery-Tab, erythromycin, Ilosone,* and *PCE.*

4. sulfonamides: *Bactrim, Gantrisin, Gantanol, Septra,* and *TMP-SMZ.*

5. fluoroquinolones: *Cipro, Floxin,* and *Noroxin.*

6. tetracyclines: *Achromycin V, Declomycin, Doryx, doxycycline, Minocin, Sumycin, tetracycline,* and *Vibramycin.*

7. *Cleocin* and *Lincocin.*

8. urinary tract anti-infectives: *Hiprex, Macrodantin, mandelamine, NegGram,* and *Urex.*

9. miscellaneous: *Augmentin, chloramphenicol, Flagyl, metronidazole, Neomycin,* and *Vancocin.*

Some antibacterial products contain more than one ingredient:

> *Augmentin* = amoxicillin + potassium clavulanate
> *Bactrim* (or *Septra*) = trimethoprim + sulfamethoxazole

## Side Effects and Drug Interactions

The one side effect common to many of the antibiotics is upset stomach, which can be minimized by taking them with food. There are a few exceptions, though—penicillin, tetracycline, and Lincocin should all be taken on an empty stomach because they are better absorbed when not combined with food.

Some antibiotics may cause *photosensitivity reactions*, that is, they may increase your susceptibility to a sunburn. If you are taking any of the tetracyclines or sulfonamides, be sure to wear a sunscreen if you plan to stay in the sun for an extended period of time.

If you are taking Flagyl (metronidazole), you should beware of the interaction between this antibiotic and alcohol. This combination may cause severe nausea and vomiting, headache, sweating, and facial flushing. Take special notice of cough medicines that may contain alcohol. If you need to take a cough medicine, ask your pharmacist to recommend one that is alcohol-free.

Finally, be sure to take your antibiotic until all of the medication is finished, unless your doctor tells you to stop early. Too often, people stop taking their antibiotics a few days early because they feel better. Stopping early can lead to bacterial resistance (and lack of effectiveness the next time you use that antibiotic) because residual bacteria (the ones that are the toughest to get rid of) may still be present, even though you feel well.

Note in the drug interaction chart that some interactions include only penicillin or tetracycline, while others cover the whole category of penicillins or tetracyclines.

## DRUG INTERACTION CHART:
## ANTIBIOTICS TO TREAT INFECTION

| Drug Interaction | Rating* | Potential Effects/Recommendations |
|---|---|---|
| Ampicillin/Zyloprim | C | See Key 26. |
| Cipro/Antacids | A | Cipro may be less effective. Do not take an antacid unless your doctor tells you to do so. If you are taking an antacid to treat an ulcer, take the antacid six hours before or two hours after Cipro. |
| Cipro/Carafate | A | Cipro may be less effective. Contact your doctor if your infection or illness has not improved after two days of Cipro therapy. |

| Drug Interaction | Rating* | Potential Effects/Recommendations |
|---|---|---|
| Cipro/Coumadin | D | See Key 19. |
| Cipro/Cytoxan | B | Cipro may be less effective. Your doctor may want to check your Cipro blood level and may adjust your dosage. |
| Cipro/Iron | A | Cipro binds with iron in the intestine and may not be absorbed into the bloodstream. Cipro may be less effective if taken with iron, so do not take iron supplements unless your doctor has told you to do so. |
| Cipro/Sandimmune | B | See Key 34. |
| Cipro/Theophylline | A | See Key 20. |
| Cipro/Zinc | C | Cipro may be less effective. Do not take zinc supplements while taking Cipro. If you are using a multivitamin that contains zinc, take the multivitamin six hours before or two hours after Cipro. |
| Erythromycin/Coumadin | C | See Key 19. |
| Erythromycin/Digoxin | B | See Key 17. |
| Erythromycin/Halcion | C | See Key 21. |
| Erythromycin/Medrol | B | See Key 29. |
| Erythromycin/Mevacor | B | See Key 18. |
| Erythromycin/Migraine Headache Medications That Contain Ergotamine | A | See Key 26. |
| Erythromycin/Norpace | B | See Key 16. |
| Erythromycin/Parlodel | B | See Key 34. |
| Erythromycin/Sandimmune | A | See Key 34. |
| Erythromycin/Tegretol | A | See Key 30. |
| Erythromycin/Theophylline | A | See Key 20. |

| Drug Interaction | Rating* | Potential Effects/Recommendations |
|---|---|---|
| Flagyl/Alcohol | A | You may experience headache, nausea, sweating, and facial flushing. It is best to avoid alcohol while taking Flagyl. Beware: many nonprescription cough medicines contain enough alcohol per dose to produce these symptoms if combined with Flagyl. |
| Flagyl/Anticoagulants | A | See Key 19. |
| Flagyl/Contac Nighttime Cold Medicine Liquid | A | See Key 39. |
| Flagyl/Dilantin | D | See Key 30. |
| Flagyl/NyQuil Nighttime Cold Medicine Liquid | A | See Key 39. |
| Flagyl/Questran | D | Flagyl may not be completely absorbed into the bloodstream and may therefore be less effective. Take Questran six hours before or two hours after Flagyl. |
| Flagyl/Terpin Hydrate Elixir | A | See Key 39. |
| Hiprex/Diamox | A | Hiprex may be less effective. If your urinary tract symptoms have not improved within two days, contact your doctor. |
| Hiprex/Sulfonamide Antibiotics | A | This combination may cause crystals to form in the urine. Do not take both medications together unless your doctor tells you to do so. |
| Macrodantin/Antacids | D | Macrodantin may be less effective if taken with antacids (or laxatives) that contain magnesium. Ask your pharmacist to help you select an antacid that does not contain magnesium. If you are taking an antacid to treat an ulcer, take the antacid several hours after Macrodantin. |
| Macrodantin/Dilantin | D | See Key 30. |

139

| Drug Interaction | Rating* | Potential Effects/Recommendations |
|---|---|---|
| Macrodantin/Food | C | Take Macrodantin with food to improve the absorption of the drug and minimize stomach upset (a common side effect of Macrodantin). |
| Mandelamine/Sulfonamides | A | This combination may cause crystals to form in the urine. Do not take both medications together unless your doctor tells you to do so. |
| NegGram/Anticoagulants | D | See Key 19. |
| Noroxin/Antacids | A | Noroxin may be less effective. Do not take an antacid unless your doctor tells you to do so. If you are taking an antacid to treat an ulcer, take the antacid six hours before or two hours after Noroxin. |
| Noroxin/Carafate | A | Noroxin may be less effective. Contact your doctor if your infection or illness has not improved after two days of Noroxin therapy. |
| Noroxin/Coumadin | D | See Key 19. |
| Noroxin/Cytoxan | B | Noroxin may be less effective. Your doctor may want to check your Noroxin blood level and may adjust your dosage. |
| Noroxin/Food | A | Noroxin may be less effective when taken with food. To minimize this interaction, take Noroxin one hour before meals. |
| Noroxin/Theophylline | A | See Key 20. |
| Penicillin/Food | A | Penicillin may be less effective if taken with food. Take penicillin on an empty stomach, one hour before or two hours after meals. |
| The Penicillins/Benemid | A | Any one of the penicillins may have a more potent effect. If you are getting a prescription for an antibiotic, be sure to tell your doctor you are taking Benemid. |

| Drug Interaction | Rating* | Potential Effects/Recommendations |
|---|---|---|
| The Penicillins/ Erythromycin | D | This interaction may occur if your doctor gives you a prescription for erythromycin to treat a chest or nasal infection, and your dentist prescribes penicillin for mitral valve protection. It is usually not necessary to take both antibiotics together; also, when they are combined, pencillin may be less effective. Contact your doctor or dentist before taking these antibiotics on the same day. |
| The Penicillins/ The Tetracyclines | A | This interaction may occur if your doctor gives you a prescription for a tetracycline type antibiotic to treat an infection, and your dentist gives you a prescription for penicillin for mitral valve protection. It is usually not necessary to take both antibiotics together, and, when combined, pencillin may be less effective. Contact your doctor or dentist before taking these antibiotics on the same day. |
| Sulfonamides/ Coumadin | A | See Key 19. |
| Sulfonamides/ Diabetes Medicines | C | See Key 28. |
| Sulfonamides/Dilantin | A | See Key 30. |
| Sulfonamides/MAOIs | B | See Key 23. |
| Sulfonamides/ Methotrexate | B | See Key 33. |
| Sulfonamides/ Sandimmune | A | See Key 34. |
| Tetracycline/Antacids | A | Tetracycline may not be absorbed and may not be effective. Take the antacid four hours before or one hour after tetracycline. |
| Tetracycline/ Anticoagulants | D | See Key 19. |

| Drug Interaction | Rating* | Potential Effects/Recommendations |
|---|---|---|
| Tetracycline/Calcium | A | Tetracycline may not be absorbed and may not be effective. Take the calcium supplement four hours before or one hour after tetracycline. |
| Tetracycline/Charcoal | A | Tetracycline may not be absorbed and may not be effective. Ask your pharmacist to help you to select an intestinal gas medication that does not contain charcoal. |
| Tetracycline/Citrate of Magnesia | A | Tetracycline may be less effective. Ask your pharmacist to recommend a laxative that does not contain magnesium. |
| Tetracycline/Digoxin | B | See Key 17. |
| Tetracycline/Food (Dairy Products) | A | Tetracycline may not be absorbed and may not be effective. Take the tetracycline one hour before or two hours after foods that contain calcium such as milk, ice cream, cheese, and other dairy products. |
| Tetracycline/Iron | A | Tetracycline may not be absorbed and may not be effective. Take the iron supplement four hours before or one hour after tetracycline. |
| Tetracycline/ Kaopectate | A | Tetracycline may not be absorbed and may not be effective. Take tetracycline one hour before or four hours after Kaopectate. |
| Tetracycline/Milk of Magnesia | A | Tetracycline may be less effective. Ask your pharmacist to recommend a laxative that does not contain magnesium. |
| Tetracycline/ Pepto-Bismol | A | Tetracycline may not be absorbed and may not be effective. Take Pepto-Bismol four hours before or one hour after tetracycline. |
| Tetracycline/TUMS | A | Tetracycline may not be completely absorbed and may therefore be less effective. Take tetracycline one hour before or three hours after TUMS. |

| Drug Interaction | Rating* | Potential Effects/Recommendations |
|---|---|---|
| Tetracycline/Zinc | A | Tetracycline may not be absorbed and may not be effective. Take the zinc supplement four hours before or one hour after tetracycline. |
| The Tetracyclines/ Colestid | D | Tetracycline, Minocin, Vibramycin, or Declomycin may not be absorbed completely. Take the antibiotic at least two hours before or after Colestid. |
| The Tetracyclines/ Insulin | D | See Key 28. |
| Vibramycin/ Anticoagulants | D | See Key 19. |
| Vibramycin/Digoxin | B | See Key 17. |
| Vibramycin/Dilantin | A | Vibramycin may be less effective when combined with Dilantin. If your infection has not improved within three days, contact your doctor. |
| Vibramycin/ Pepto-Bismol | A | You may have heard about this combination to prevent traveler's diarrhea. However, Vibramycin may not be completely absorbed if taken with Pepto-Bismol at the same time. Take Vibramycin one hour before or four hours after Pepto-Bismol. |

* The rating indicates how harmful a drug interaction may be and how frequently it may occur.

"A" indicates a drug interaction that may cause serious harm and occurs frequently. "B" indicates a drug interaction that may cause serious harm but occurs less frequently. "C" indicates a drug interaction that is less harmful but occurs frequently. "D" indicates a drug interaction that is less harmful and occurs less frequently. See Key 9 for more information about the rating system.

# 32

# OTHER MEDICATIONS PRESCRIBED FOR INFECTIONS

In this Key we will focus mainly on the medications prescribed for infections that are not caused by bacteria. Fungus infections (including *Candida* infections) and viruses cannot be cured with antibiotics. Each of these "living pests" must be eradicated with its own type of medication. Tuberculosis (TB) is also discussed in this Key because it is caused by an unusual form of bacteria.

In the antifungal category, Nystatin is most often prescribed to treat *Candida* infections in the mouth (thrush) and intestinal tract. Fulvicin (Grisactin) is the favorite for fungal nail infections; Nizoral is also prescribed for fungal nail and skin infections, as well as fungal infections in the blood. Diflucan is usually reserved for people at high risk for developing life-threatening fungal infections, such as persons who have cancer or AIDS).

In the antiviral category, Symmetrel (amantadine) is most often prescribed to prevent a full-blown influenza A viral infection. Zovirax is used to treat herpes simplex viruses, and Retrovir is prescribed for HIV, the virus associated with AIDS. However, neither Zovirax or Retrovir actually cures the infections.

The treatment for tuberculosis usually consists of a combination of several medications.

### The Medications

The antifungal medications are *Diflucan, Fulvicin, Grisactin, Nizoral,* and *Nystatin.*

The antiviral medications are *amantadine, Retrovir, Symmetrel,* and *Zovirax.*

The tuberculosis medications are *isoniazid (INH), rifampin,* and *para-aminosalicylic acid (PAS).*

## Side Effects and Drug Interactions

### Antifungals

The most common side effect of the antifungal drugs is stomach upset, which may be minimized by taking them with food. In fact, Fulvicin (Grisactin) is better absorbed when it is taken with food—a desirable effect.

Nizoral requires stomach acid to dissolve and disintegrate so that it can be absorbed into the bloodstream. Other medications may interfere with Nizoral's absorption (and subsequent effectiveness) by reducing the amount of acid in the stomach. Antacids neutralize stomach acid, and ulcer medications, such as Axid, Tagamet, Zantac, and Pepcid, reduce the amount of acid secreted in the stomach. To minimize the effects of this drug interaction, take Nizoral at least two hours before antacids, and one hour before the ulcer medications.

### Antivirals

The most common side effects of Symmetrel (amantadine) are dizziness, nausea, and insomnia. It may interfere with other medications, but Symmetrel itself is usually not affected.

Since Retrovir may cause blood abnormalities, your doctor may want you to get blood counts regularly. Zovirax is generally well tolerated; nausea and headache seem to be the most common side effects.

### Tuberculosis Medications

Rifampin and isoniazid (INH) interact with other drugs by changing their metabolism. Rifampin increases the metabolism of some drugs, causing them to be eliminated from the body faster than they should be. The result may be reduced effectiveness or ineffectiveness of the other medication.

INH has been shown to increase or decrease the metabolism of other drugs, and this may affect *their* potency. Unfortunately, you cannot prevent these types of interactions by taking the medications a few hours apart. Therefore, your doctor may want to adjust the dosage of your medications.

## DRUG INTERACTION CHART:
## OTHER MEDICATIONS PRESCRIBED
## FOR INFECTIONS

| Drug Interaction | Rating* | Potential Effects/Recommendations |
|---|---|---|
| Diflucan/Rifampin | B | Diflucan may be less effective. Your doctor may adjust your Diflucan dosage. |
| Fulvicin/Coumadin | D | See Key 19. |
| Fulvicin/Food | C | It is best to take Fulvicin with food (that is, immediately after a meal) to improve its absorption into the blood stream and to minimize stomach upset—a common side effect of this drug. |
| Fulvicin/Mysoline | D | Fulvicin may be less effective. Your doctor may adjust your Fulvicin dosage. |
| Fulvicin/Phenobarbital | D | Fulvicin may be less effective. Your doctor may adjust your Fulvicin dosage. |
| Isoniazid (INH)/Alcohol | C | If you drink alcoholic beverages every day while taking INH, you are at increased risk for developing liver impairment or hepatitis. Ask your doctor whether you may drink alcoholic beverages and, if so, what quantity what is safe. |
| Isoniazid (INH)/ Antacids | D | INH may not be completely absorbed into the bloodstream and may be less effective. Take INH at least two hours before the antacid. |
| Isoniazid (INH)/ Anticoagulants | D | See Key 19. |
| Isoniazid (INH)/ Benzodiazepines | D | See Key 21. |

146

| Drug Interaction | Rating* | Potential Effects/Recommendations |
|---|---|---|
| Isoniazid (INH)/ Dilantin | A | See Key 30. |
| Isoniazid (INH)/Food | C | INH may be less effective if taken with food. The combination of INH and some cheeses may cause headache, chills, and facial flushing. It is best to take INH one hour before, or two hours after meals. |
| Isoniazid (INH)/ Mysoline | D | See Key 22. |
| Isonizide (INH)/ Rifampin | B | Some people may be at increased risk of developing liver impairment. Your doctor may want to check your liver function while you are taking this drug combination. |
| Isoniazid (INH)/ Tegretol | A | See Key 30. |
| Isoniazid (INH)/ Theophylline | C | See Key 20. |
| Nizoral/Alcohol | C | You may experience headache, chills and facial flushing. It is best to avoid alcoholic beverages while taking Nizoral. |
| Nizoral/Antacids | D | Nizoral may be less effective if taken immediately after an antacid. Take Nizoral at least two hours before the antacid to minimize this interaction. |
| Nizoral/Axid | D | Nizoral may be less effective because it requires stomach acid to dissolve and then be absorbed. Since Axid reduces stomach acid, you should take Nizoral one hour before Axid to minimize this drug interaction. |
| Nizoral/Corticosteroids | A | See Key 29. |
| Nizoral/Coumadin | B | See Key 19. |

147

| Drug Interaction | Rating* | Potential Effects/Recommendations |
|---|---|---|
| Nizoral/Isoniazid (INH) | B | Nizoral may be less effective. Your doctor may want to examine your fungal infection regularly to be sure that it is improving. |
| Nizoral/Pepcid | D | Nizoral may be less effective because it requires stomach acid to dissolve and then be absorbed. Because Pepcid reduces stomach acid, you should take Nizoral one hour before Pepcid to minimize this drug interaction. |
| Nizoral/Rifampin | A | Both Nizoral and rifampin may be less effective. Your doctor may adjust the dosages of both drugs. |
| Nizoral/Seldane | A | See Key 27. |
| Nizoral/Tagamet | D | Nizoral may be less effective because it requires stomach acid to dissolve and then be absorbed. Since Tagamet reduces stomach acid, you should take Nizoral one hour before Tagamet to minimize this drug interaction. |
| Nizoral/Theophylline | D | See Key 20. |
| Nizoral/Zantac | D | Nizoral may be less effective because it requires stomach acid to dissolve and then be absorbed. Because Zantac reduces stomach acid, you should take Nizoral one hour before Zantac to minimize this drug interaction. |
| Retrovir/Benemid | A | Retrovir may have a more potent action. This combination is sometimes prescribed to reduce the number of daily dosages required for treatment. If you experience such side effects as skin rash, or fever with aches and pains, contact your doctor *right away*. |
| Retrovir/Food | A | Retrovir may be less effective if taken immediately after a high-fat meal. Take Retrovir one hour before or two hours after your meals. |

| Drug Interaction | Rating* | Potential Effects/Recommendations |
|---|---|---|
| Rifampin/ Anticoagulants | A | See Key 19. |
| Rifampin/ Benzodiazepines | D | See Key 21. |
| Rifampin/ Beta Blockers | A | See Key 14. |
| Rifampin/ Corticosteroids | A | See Key 29. |
| Rifampin/Diabetes Medicines | C | See Key 28. |
| Rifampin/Digoxin | B | See Key 17. |
| Rifampin/Dilantin | A | See Key 30. |
| Rifampin/Haldol | D | See Key 24. |
| Rifampin/Norpace | A | See Key 16. |
| Rifampin/Quinindine | A | See Key 16. |
| Rifampin/Sandimmune | A | See Key 34. |
| Rifampin/ Theophylline | A | See Key 20. |
| Rifampin/Vasotec | B | See Key 12. |
| Symmetrel/Artane | C | See Key 34. |
| Symmetrel/Cogentin | C | See Key 34. |
| Zovirax/Retrovir | D | You may feel lethargic or fatigued. If you experience these symptoms, tell your doctor. |

* The rating indicates how harmful a drug interaction may be and how frequently it may occur.

"A" indicates a drug interaction that may cause serious harm and occurs frequently. "B" indicates a drug interaction that may cause serious harm but occurs less frequently. "C" indicates a drug interaction that is less harmful but occurs frequently. "D" indicates a drug interaction that is less harmful and occurs less frequently. See Key 9 for more information about the rating system.

# 33

## MEDICATIONS TO TREAT CANCER

*Cancer* is a disease in which abnormal cells of a tissue or organ grow in an uncontrollable manner. Normal cells replicate and die; there is a balance between the number of cells that die and the number of new cells that replace them. In contrast, cancerous cells replicate very quickly—more quickly than do normal cells. By their sheer numbers, the cancerous cells overwhelm the normal cells and basically "steal" their nutrition.

Cancer medications act by "seeking out" the fastest growing cells and killing them. Unfortunately, certain types of normal cells, such as hair follicle cells and the mucous membrane cells that line the gastrointestinal tract, also grow rapidly and may become unintended targets of the drug. This is the reason that people who have *chemotherapy* (a certain class of cancer medication) tend to lose their hair and may experience ulcers in the mouth and throat *(stomatitis)*.

### The Medications

The most commonly prescribed oral cancer medications are as follows:

1. alkylating agents: *Alkeran, CeeNu, Cytoxan, Leukeran,* and *Myleran.*
2. antimetabolites: *methotrexate,* and *Purinethol.*
3. *Nolvadex.*
4. *Matulane.*
5. *Cytadren.*

Methotrexate is also used in the treatment of severe rheumatoid arthritis, and severe cases of psoriasis.

## Side Effects and Drug Interactions

The side effects of cancer medications are probably the most severe of any category of drugs. Depending on the individual medication, a person getting chemotherapy may experience nausea, vomiting, diarrhea, aches and pains, fever, chills, ulcers in the mouth, hair loss, blood abnormalities, and reduced resistance to infections.

If the side effects of cancer medications are so severe, isn't it better not to take them? In most cases, no. After all, many cancers are potentially fatal, and these medications have prolonged and saved lives.

New cancer treatments are being discovered every year. Also, with better technology, cancers are being detected early, before they've become too extensive, thereby increasing the chance of survival. Your doctor will probably tell you that in most cases the benefit of the medications (that is, the chance to save your life) outweighs the risks (the side effects of the drugs).

## DRUG INTERACTION CHART:
## MEDICATIONS TO TREAT CANCER

| Drug Interaction | Rating* | Potential Effects/Recommendations |
|---|---|---|
| Cytoxan/Cipro | B | See Key 31. |
| Cytoxan/Coumadin | D | See Key 19. |
| Cytoxan/Noroxin | B | See Key 31. |
| Cytoxan/Zyloprim | D | Cytoxan may have a slightly more potent effect. Be sure to keep your appointments for blood tests. |
| Methotrexate/Alcohol | B | This combination may increase the risk of liver dysfunction. Ask your doctor whether you can drink alcoholic beverages with methotrexate. |

| Drug Interaction | Rating* | Potential Effects/Recommendations |
|---|---|---|
| Methotrexate/Aspirin | C | Methotrexate may have a more potent action. Ask your doctor whether you can take aspirin with methotrexate and, if so, what dosage is correct. Before purchasing a nonprescription pain reliever, ask your pharmacist whether the product contains aspirin or any aspirinlike ingredients. |
| Methotrexate/Benemid | A | Methotrexate may have a more potent action. Your doctor may adjust your dosage. Be sure to keep appointments for blood tests. |
| Methotrexate/Butazolidin | A | Methotrexate may have a more potent effect. If you experience such side effects as fever and ulceration of the mouth or skin, contact your doctor. |
| Methotrexate/Charcoal | A | Methotrexate may be less effective. Ask your pharmacist to suggest an intestinal gas medication that does not contain charcoal. |
| Methotrexate/Digoxin | B | See Key 17. |
| Methotrexate/Dilantin | A | See Key 30. |
| Methotrexate/NSAIDs | A | Methotrexate may have a more potent effect, especially when taken with Indocin. Do not combine a nonprescription medication (such as ibuprofen) and methotrexate without first asking your doctor. |
| Methotrexate/Pepto-Bismol | A | Methotrexate may have a more potent effect. The active ingredient of Pepto-Bismol is a member of the salicylate family of medications, which retard the elimination of methotrexate from the body. Ask your pharmacist to help you select an antidiarrheal medicine that does not contain bismuth subsalicylate. |

| Drug Interaction | Rating* | Potential Effects/Recommendations |
|---|---|---|
| Methotrexate/Questran | A | Methotrexate may be less effective because it binds with Questran in the intestinal tract and is not completely absorbed. Take your methotrexate and Questran dosages several hours apart. |
| Methotrexate/ Salicylates | A | Methotrexate may have a more potent effect. Ask your pharmacist to recommend a pain reliever that does not contain a salicylate. |
| Methotrexate/ Sulfonamides | B | This combination may increase the risk of methotrexate side effects involving blood cells. Be sure to keep appointments for blood tests. |
| Nolvadex/Coumadin | B | See Key 19. |

* The rating indicates how harmful a drug interaction may be and how frequently it may occur.

"A" indicates a drug interaction that may cause serious harm and occurs frequently. "B" indicates a drug interaction that may cause serious harm but occurs less frequently. "C" indicates a drug interaction that is less harmful but occurs frequently. "D" indicates a drug interaction that is less harmful and occurs less frequently. See Key 9 for more information about the rating system.

# 34

## MISCELLANEOUS PRESCRIPTION DRUG INTERACTIONS

Within this grab bag of prescription medications, we will focus on medications prescribed for *Parkinson's disease* and those related to *organ transplant rejection.*

Parkinson's disease may be described as a nerve disorder resulting in muscle rigidity, tremor, and increased difficulty in movement, particularly in walking, chewing, swallowing, and speaking.

Psychiatric medications sometimes cause Parkinson-like side effects, which may be minimized with the use of Artane or Cogentin. In fact, Haldol and Cogentin are prescribed together quite often.

### The Medications

Some medications used for Parkinson's disease are as follows:

1. anticholinergics: *Artane, benztropine, Cogentin,* and *trihexyphenidyl.*
2. dopaminergics: *Eldepryl, levodopa, Parlodel, Sinemet* (= levodopa + carbidopa), and *Symmetrel* (see Key 32).

Two immunosuppressive drugs that prevent tissue rejection from organ transplants are *Imuran* and *Sandimmune.*

### Side Effects and Drug Interactions

**Medications for Parkinson's Disease**

The most common side effects of the anticholinergic drugs are dizziness, drowsiness, blurred vision, and dry mouth. These side effects may become more pronounced if other medications increase the potency of Artane or Cogentin.

154

The most common side effects of levodopa and other dopaminergics are abnormal movements, nausea, vomiting, anorexia, loss of taste, weakness, dizziness, headache, and mood changes. These side effects may become more pronounced if another medication increases the potency of levodopa or Sinemet. On the other hand, other drugs may reduce the effectiveness of levodopa or Sinemet and thereby worsen the Parkinson's symptoms.

Parlodel is generally well tolerated, but when combined with other medications that may increase its potency, side effects such as nausea, confusion, and involuntary movements may occur.

## Immunosuppressive Drugs

The most serious side effects of both Imuran and Sandiummune are blood abnormalities. If you are taking either of these medications, your doctor will probably want to check your blood count regularly. This precautionary measure is important, so be sure to keep your appointments for blood work.

Other side effects of Sandimmune are reduced kidney function, high blood pressure, tremor, extra hair growth, increased size of the gums, and increased susceptiblity to infection.

Side effects are more likely to occur if your Sandimmune blood level (the amount in the blood) gets too high. Conversely, if your Sandimmune blood level is too low, the drug may not be effective, and you may be at increased risk for organ rejection. To ensure that your dosage is correct, your doctor may want to check your Sandimmune blood level and, as a precaution, your kidney function on a regular basis.

# DRUG INTERACTION CHART: MISCELLANEOUS
# PRESCRIPTION DRUG INTERACTIONS

| Drug Interaction | Rating | Potential Effects/Recommendations |
|---|---|---|
| Artane/Symmetrel | C | Artane may have a more potent effect. If you experience blurred vision, dry mouth, dizziness, and drowsiness, contact your doctor. Your Artane dosage may have to be adjusted. |
| Cogentin/Symmetrel | C | Cogentin may have a more potent effect. If you experience blurred vision, dry mouth, dizziness and drowsiness, contact your doctor. Your Cogentin dosage may have to be adjusted. |
| Imuran/Zyloprim | A | Immuran may have a more potent effect. Your doctor may adjust your Immuran dosage. Immuran can reduce your white blood cell count, so be sure to keep your appointments with the lab for blood tests. |
| Levodopa/Antispasmodics | B | You may experience levodopa side effects (involuntary muscle movements, mood changes). Your doctor may adjust your levodopa dosage. |
| Levodopa/Dilantin | A | Levodopa may be less effective. Your doctor may adjust your levodopa dosage. |
| Levodopa/Iron | C | Levodopa may bind with iron in the intestinal tract and may not be completely absorbed. Therefore, levodopa may be less effective. To minimize this interaction, take iron supplements two hours before or after levodopa. (Multivitamins that contain small amounts of iron are less likely to interact with levodopa and can be taken at any time.) |
| Levodopa/MAOIS | A | See Key 23. |
| Levodopa/Reglan | B | You may experience levodopa side effects (involuntary muscle movements, mood changes). Your doctor may adjust your levodopa dosage. |

| Drug Interaction | Rating* | Potential Effects/Recommendations |
|---|---|---|
| Levodopa/TCAs | D | Levodopa may be less effective. If your Parkison's disease symptoms worsen, contact your doctor. Your levodopa dosage may need to be adjusted. |
| Levodopa/Vitamin B$_6$ | A | Levodopa may be less effective. However, if you are taking Sinemet, a product that also contains carbidopa, this interaction is unlikely to occur. |
| Parlodel/Alcohol | B | Parlodel may have a more potent effect. Ask your doctor whether you may drink alcoholic beverages with Parlodel and, if so, what quantity is safe. This combination can cause nausea, confusion, and increased involuntary muscle movements. If you develop these symptoms, contact your doctor. |
| Parlodel/Erythromycin | B | Parlodel may have a more potent effect which can lead to side effects such as nausea, confusion, and involuntary muscle movements. If these symptoms occur, contact your doctor. |
| Sandimmune/CCBs | A | Sandimmune may have a more potent effect, which may affect the kidneys. Your doctor may want to check your Sandimmune blood level and kidney function regularly. |
| Sandimmune/Cipro | B | This combination may increase the risk of reduced kidney function. Your doctor may want to check your kidney function while you are taking Cipro. |
| Sandimmune/ Corticosteroids | B | See Key 29. |
| Sandimmune/Digoxin | A | See Key 17. |
| Sandimmune/Dilantin | A | Sandimmune may be less effective. Your doctor may want to check your Sandimmune blood level if your Dilantin dosage changes. Do not skip doses of either medication. |

| Drug Interaction | Rating* | Potential Effects/Recommendations |
|---|---|---|
| Sandimmune/ Erythromycin | A | Sandimmune may have a more potent effect, which may affect the kidneys. Your doctor may want to check your Sandimmune blood level and kidney function regularly. |
| Sandimmune/Mevacor | A | See Key 18. |
| Sandimmune/Nizoral | A | Sandimmune may have a more potent effect, which may affect the kidneys. Your doctor may want to check your Sandimmune blood level and kidney function regularly. |
| Sandimmune/Reglan | B | You may experience such side effects as headache, tremor, fever, and fatigue. If you do, contact your doctor. The Sandimmune dosage may have to be adjusted. |
| Sandimmune/Rifampin | A | Sandimmune may be less effective. Your doctor may check your Sandimmune blood level, and may adjust your dosage. |
| Sandimmune/ Sulfonamides | A | Sandimmune may be less effective. In addition, this combination may increase the risk of reduced kidney function. Your doctor may want to check your Sandimmune blood level and kidney fuction while you are taking sulfonamide antibiotics. |

* The rating indicates how harmful a drug interaction may be and how frequently it may occur.

"A" indicates a drug interaction that may cause serious harm and occurs frequently. "B" indicates a drug interaction that may cause serious harm but occurs less frequently. "C" indicates a drug interaction that is less harmful but occurs frequently. "D" indicates a drug interaction that is less harmful and occurs less frequently. See Key 9 for more information about the rating system.

# 35

## ASPIRIN AND OTHER NONPRESCRIPTION PAIN RELIEVERS

It always amazes me when I peek down the aisle marked "Pain Relievers" in the pharmacy or supermarket. There may be fifteen or twenty shelves stocked with these products! Actually, however, there are only three kinds of pain medications you can buy without a prescription (see below).

As you have probably guessed, manufacturers are very creative in the way they package and market their products. Some may add an extra ingredient, such as caffeine, just to make their products different. Others try to invent a new way to take the medication. (Who ever heard of bubbling aspirin? Obviously, the makers of Alka-Seltzer did.)

One of the biggest controversies of the early 1980s involved the concept of generic drugs. I'll bet that the first time you reached for the "less expensive brand" you took a moment to reconsider and ended up walking out with the brand-name product. "When it comes to medicine," people would tell me, "I want the best!" Nowadays, things are different. Instead of asking which aisle the Advil, Nuprin, or Medipren is in, people simply inquire, "Where's the ibuprofen?"

### The Medications

As stated above, there are three categories of nonprescription pain relievers:

1. acetaminophen: *Anacin-3, Datril, Panadol, Tempra,* and *Tylenol.*
2. ibuprofen: *Advil, Medipren, Motrin IB, Nuprin,* and *Pamprin IB.*

3. salicylates: *Arthropan, aspirin, Doan's Pills*, and salicylates found in rubs and liniments (*Ben-Gay* and *Icy-Hot*). Aspirin comes in many different forms: tablets (*Bayer* and many other brands), enteric-coated tablets *(Ecotrin)*, buffered tablets *(Bufferin)*, effervescent tablets (*Alka-Seltzer*, Flavored), timed release tablets *(Measurin)*, chewing gum *(Aspergum)*, and suppositories.

You may be surprised at what ingredients are in some of the most popular pain relief products. Here is a small sampling:

*Anacin* = aspirin + caffeine

*Ascriptin* = aspirin + magnesium and aluminum hydroxides, and calcium carbonate (antacids)

*Bufferin Extra-Strength* = aspirin + magnesium carbonate + aluminum glycinate (buffers)

*Excedrin* = acetaminophen + aspirin + caffeine

*Momentum Caplets* = aspirin + phenyltoloxamine (an antihistamine)

*Vanquish Caplets* = acetaminophen + aspirin + caffeine + magnesium and aluminum hydroxides (antacids)

Which pain reliever is the best? The answer depends on the condition you are treating. All three categories reduce fever; however, ibuprofen may be more effective for high fevers (over 102.5°F).

All three relieve mild aches and pain. Only aspirin and ibuprofen, however, relieve rheumatoid arthritis pain because they reduce inflammation, whereas acetaminophen does not.

## Side Effects and Drug Interactions

### Salicylates

Aspirin may cause upset stomach and nausea but these can be minimized by taking aspirin tablets that are coated or buffered. A more serious side effect that may occur is bleeding in the intestinal tract, which can lead to ulcers *in persons susceptible to them.* If you have ever had an ulcer, it is a good idea to stay away from aspirin.

The arthritis dosage of aspirin is much higher than the regular dosage to treat fever or minor aches and pains. If you are taking large doses of aspirin, you should be aware of a warning sign that may indicate you've had too much: ringing in the ears. If you experience this symptom, contact your doctor right away.

If you take aspirin, make sure you do not take other drug products that also contain aspirin or other salicylates, such as Pepto-Bismol, at the same time. When these drugs are combined, you may experience side effects (for example, ringing in the ears).

Topical rubs or liniments such as Ben-Gay or Icy-Hot also contain salicylates. Do not apply these products to open wounds, and do not use too much at one time—the salicylates in these products may be absorbed through the skin, into the bloodstream. If you combine these rubs or liniments with high doses of aspirin taken orally, you may experience aspirin side effects.

Acetaminophen and ibuprofen are more gentle on the stomach than aspirin. Nevertheless, ibuprofen may cause stomach upset and should therefore be taken with food. Acetaminophen is well tolerated and rarely causes side effects. It does not tend to cause stomach upset and is compatible with most other medications.

## DRUG INTERACTION CHART:
## ASPIRIN AND OTHER NONPRESCRIPTION
## PAIN RELIEVERS

| Drug Interaction | Rating* | Potential Effects/Recommendations |
|---|---|---|
| Acetaminophen/ Alcohol | C | If you drink alcoholic beverages and take acetaminophen every day, you may be at increased risk for developing liver abnormalities. Avoid daily use of alcohol and acetaminophen. (Occasional use of this combination will not increase this risk.) |

| Drug Interaction | Rating* | Potential Effects/Recommendations |
|---|---|---|
| Acetaminophen/ Charcoal | C | Acetaminophen may not be absorbed and may be less effective. Ask your pharmacist to help you select another medication to relieve intestinal gas. |
| Acetaminophen/ Questran | C | Acetaminophen may not be absorbed and may be less effective. Take acetaminophen one hour before or several hours after Questran. |
| Aspirin/ACE Inhibitors | D | See Key 12. |
| Aspirin/Alcohol | B | This combination may increase the risk of intestinal bleeding *in some people*. If you have a history of ulcers, do not combine aspirin with alcohol. In fact, it is a good idea not to use aspirin or alcohol if you have an ulcer. |
| Aspirin/Antacids | C | Aspirin may be less effective if you take large doses of antacids. |
| Aspirin/Anticoagulants | A | See Key 19. |
| Aspirin/Axid | D | Aspirin may have a more potent effect. If you are taking large doses of aspirin every day (eight 500-mg or twelve 325-mg tablets), you may experience aspirin side effects, such as ringing in the ears, when you start taking Axid. Your doctor may adjust your aspirin dosage. |
| Aspirin/Corticosteroids | A | This combination may cause upset stomach. Take both medications with food. Aspirin may be less effective for those who take large amounts and then start taking a corticosteroid. If your aspirin seems to have lost its effective-ness, do not take more without first consulting your doctor. |
| Aspirin/Depakene | A | See Key 30. |
| Aspirin/Diabetes Medicines | A | See Key 28. |

| Drug Interaction | Rating* | Potential Effects/Recommendations |
|---|---|---|
| Aspirin/Diamox | A | See Key 13. |
| Aspirin/Insulin | A | See Key 28. |
| Aspirin/Methotrexate | C | See Key 33. |
| Aspirin/Nitroglycerin | D | See Key 15. |
| Aspirin/Pepto-Bismol | C | Both medications are salicylates. This combination may increase the risk of salicylate side effects, such as ringing in the ears. If this happens to you, stop taking both drugs and contact your doctor. |
| Ibuprofen/ Anticoagulants | D | See Key 19. |
| Ibuprofen/Beta Blockers | C | See Key 14. |
| Ibuprofen/Digoxin | D | See Key 17. |
| Ibuprofen/Lasix | D | See Key 13. |
| Salicylates (Including Aspirin)/Anturane | A | See Key 26. |
| Salicylates (Including Aspirin)/Benemid | A | See Key 26. |
| Salicylates/Diabetes Medicines | A | See Key 28. |
| Salicylates/ Pepto-Bismol | C | *Drug duplication:* although not used as a pain reliever, Pepto-Bismol is a member of the salicylate family and should not be taken simultaneously with other drug products that contain large doses of salicylates. To be safe, take aspirin or other salicylate drug products four hours before or after Pepto-Bismol. |

* The rating indicates how harmful a drug interaction may be and how frequently it may occur.

"A" indicates a drug interaction that may cause serious harm and occurs frequently. "B" indicates a drug interaction that may cause serious harm but occurs less frequently. "C" indicates a drug interaction that is less harmful but occurs frequently. "D" indicates a drug interaction that is less harmful and occurs less frequently. See Key 9 for more information about the rating system.

# 36

# ANTACIDS

"Plop plop, fizz fizz—Oh, what a relief it is!" Well said by the makers of Alka-Seltzer. Anyone who has ever experienced ulcers or even a mild case of heartburn knows how painful excess acid can be. Fortunately, *antacids* tend to work within minutes to stop the burning sensation caused by excess acid.

What is an *antacid*, anyway? It's a mediation that neutralizes acid. I'm sure you knew that, but what you may not know is that antacids are made up of two parts:

1. the *base* (such as hydroxide, carbonate, or bicarbonate), which combines with acid to neutralize it.
2. the *salt* (such as magnesium, aluminum, or calcium), which is chemically attached to the base.

In the presence of acid, the base and the salt detach from each other so that the base is free to neutralize the acid.

It is important to know this because the side effects that may be caused by a particular antacid are usually due to the salt, not the base. Therefore, if you decide to switch antacids because of an annoying side effect, you will want to find an antacid that contains a different salt. For example, if you tend to become constipated, you will probably not want to choose an antacid that contains only aluminum hydroxide because aluminum may cause constipation.

## The Medications

The antacids may be divided into those that contain:

1. aluminum: *Alternagel, Amphogel, Basaljel, Dialume, Phosphaljel,* and *Rolaids.*
2. magnesium: *Mag-Ox, Milk of Magnesia.*
3. magaldrate, an ingredient made up of *chemically combined* aluminum and magnesium antacids: *Riopan.*

4. calcium: *Alka-Mints, Equilet, Rolaids Calcium Rich, TUMS.*
5. sodium bicarbonate.

All of these products contain only one antacid. Here are some products that contain two or more antacids:

*Alka-Seltzer* = sodium bicarbonate + potassium bicarbonate + citric acid

*Camalox Tablets* = magnesium hydroxide + aluminum hydroxide + calcium carbonate

*Di-Gel Liquid* = magnesium hydroxide + aluminum hydroxide + simethicone (for intestinal gas)

*Gelusil Liquid* = magnesium hydroxide + aluminum hydroxide + simethicone (for intestinal gas)

*Maalox Suspension* = magnesium hydroxide + aluminum hydroxide

*Mylanta Liquid* = magnesium hydroxide + aluminum hydroxide + simethicone (for intestinal gas)

*Riopan Plus Suspension* = magaldrate + simethicone (for intestinal gas)

*Titralac Tablets* = calcium carbonate + glycine

### Side Effects and Drug Interactions

Antacids are usually well-tolerated. A preference for one over the other will depend mostly on which one tastes the best and which potentially bothersome side effects you want to avoid. For example, if you have high blood pressure and you are limiting your salt intake, you will probably want to avoid antacids that contain sodium (as in sodium bicarbonate).

Antacids that contain magnesium may cause loose stools or diarrhea. In fact, Milk of Magnesia is used as a laxative in higher dosages. Aluminum-containing antacids, on the other hand, may cause constipation. Therefore, if you are constipated or have hemorrhoids, you may want to avoid antacids that contain only aluminum. Many products contain mixtures of magnesium and aluminum salts, which are less likely to have any effect on the bowels.

165

Recently, antacids such as TUMS that contain calcium have been getting a great deal of publicity. "Not only can you reduce stomach acid and upset, but also meet the RDA for calcium in just one dose!" Antacids that contain calcium may offer an advantage for women who need to take a calcium supplement every day, especially those who have a family history of osteoporosis. But don't overdo it. Too much calcium carbonate may lead to side effects.

Antacids interact with many drugs, thereby preventing their absorption into the bloodstream. The drugs may bind to the antacid or may not be able to dissolve completely without enough acid. In either case, the entire dose may not be absorbed, resulting in loss of effectiveness. To minimize drug interactions between your antacid and other medications, take the other medications one to two hours before the antacid.

### DRUG INTERACTION CHART:
### ANTACIDS

| Drug Interaction | Rating* | Potential Effects/Recommendations |
| --- | --- | --- |
| Antacids/Beta Blockers | D | See Key 14. |
| Antacids/Cipro | A | See Key 31. |
| Antacids/Cotazyme | C | See Key 11. |
| Antacids/Decadron | D | See Key 29. |
| Antacids/Depakene | D | See Key 30. |
| Antacids/Digoxin | C | See Key 17. |
| Antacids/Dilantin | D | See Key 30. |
| Antacids/Iron | C | See Key 41. |
| Antacids/Isoniazid (INH) | D | See Key 32. |
| Antacids/Nizoral | D | See Key 32. |
| Antacids/Noroxin | A | See Key 31. |
| Antacids/Pancrease | C | See Key 11. |
| Antacids/Quinidine | A | See Key 16. |
| Antacids/Salicylates | D | See Key 26. |

| Drug Interaction | Rating* | Potential Effects/Recommendations |
|---|---|---|
| Antacids/Tagamet | D | See Key 10. |
| Antacids/Tetracycline | A | See Key 31. |
| Antacids/Thorazine | D | See Key 24. |
| Antacids/Viokase | C | See Key 11. |
| Antacids/Zyloprim | C | See Key 26. |
| TUMS/CCBs | C | See Key 15. |
| TUMS/Calcium Supplements | A | See Key 41. |
| TUMS/Tetracycline | A | See Key 31. |
| TUMS/Thiazides | B | This combination may lead to excessive calcium in the blood. Ask your pharmacist to help you select an antacid that does not contain calcium. |

\* The rating indicates how harmful a drug interaction may be and how frequently it may occur.

"A" indicates a drug interaction that may cause serious harm and occurs frequently. "B" indicates a drug interaction that may cause serious harm but occurs less frequently. "C" indicates a drug interaction that is less harmful but occurs frequently. "D" indicates a drug interaction that is less harmful and occurs less frequently. See Key 9 for more information about the rating system.

# 37

## MEDICATIONS TO TREAT DIARRHEA/CONSTIPATION/ INTESTINAL GAS

*Diarrhea* may be caused by several kinds of illnesses and disorders such as irritable bowel syndrome, malabsorption syndrome, lactose intolerance, and gastrointestinal infections. Abdominal cramping and intestinal gas usually accompany diarrhea. People who have diarrhea over long periods of time may become dehydrated and lose minerals that are important for the body to function properly.

*Constipation* is very common in older people because the natural movement of the intestinal walls, which pushes the stool through the intestinal tract, tends to slow down as we age. Divirticulitis and intestinal obstruction are among the other causes.

*Intestinal gas* may be caused by eating certain kinds of foods, by swallowing air, and by disorders such as malabsorption syndrome and lactose intolerance.

### The Medications

Nonprescription medications for diarrhea are as follows:
1. *Immodium AD*.
2. *Kaopectate* (kaolin-pectin) and *Donnagel*.
3. *Pepto-Bismol*.
4. *Diasorb*.

Nonprescription medications for constipation are as follows:
1. bulk laxatives: *Citrucel, Effer-Syllium, Equalactin, Fiberall, Hydrocil, Konsyl, Maltsupex, Metamucil, Serutan,* and *Unifiber*.

2. lubricant laxatives: *Agoral Plain, Kondremul Plain,* and *Mineral Oil.*
3. saline laxatives: *Citrate of Magnesia, Fleet Phospho-soda,* and *Milk of Magnesia.*
4. stimulant laxatives: *cascara, castor oil, Ducolax, Ex-Lax, Feen-a-mint, Fletcher's Castoria, Fleet Laxative,* and *Senokot.*
5. stool softeners: *Colace, Dialose, docusate sodium,* and *Surfak.*
6. suppositories: *Ducolax* and *glycerin.*
7. enemas: *Fleet, Fleet Bisacodyl,* and *Fleet Mineral Oil.*
8. combination stool softener and laxative: *Correctol, Doxidan, Peri-Colace,* and *Senekot-S.*

Two nonprescription medications used to relieve intestinal gas are as follows:
1. simethicone: *Gas-X, Mylicon,* and *Phazyme.*
2. charcoal: *Charcocaps.*

### Side Effects and Drug Interactions

**Medications for Diarrhea**

Immodium AD, once available only by prescription, is usually well tolerated but may cause dizziness, drowsiness, and dry mouth.

Pepto-Bismol is chemically similar to aspirin and may produce aspirin side effects, such as ringing in the ears, if taken in high doses, or with other drug products that contain aspirin or other salicylates.

Kaopectate acts by adhering to loose stool so that it is not free to cause symptoms—an action known as *ad*sorption. Unfortunately, other medications can also be *ad*sorbed by Kaopectate; this means that they may not be completely *ab*sorbed into the bloodstream and may be less effective.

Diarrhea may be a symptom of a more serious illness, especially if it lasts for more than a few days. Therefore, if your diarrhea does not improve within a short period of time, contact your doctor.

## Medications for Constipation

The bulk laxatives are considered to be the safest type. However, you must take them with plenty of water; otherwise, they may swell and become hardened in the intestinal tract, thereby creating an obstruction.

The lubricant laxatives contain mineral oil, which may reduce the absorption of vitamin A and possibly other fat soluble vitamins.

The saline laxatives may affect the delicate balance of fluid and electrolytes in the bloodstream. Some contain large amounts of sodium per dose. Therefore, if you have high blood pressure or are restricting your sodium intake, you should avoid these laxatives.

The stimulant laxatives act directly on the wall of the intestine to push the stool through the intestinal tract. These laxatives tend to have a stronger effect than the others. However, if you use them repeatedly over long periods of time, you may have difficulty passing stools when you stop taking them.

Stool softeners act by drawing water and fat into the stool, making it softer and easier to pass. Stool softeners are usually well-tolerated.

## Medications for Intestinal Gas

Simethicone acts by breaking up gas bubbles in the intestinal tract. It is effective, well-tolerated, and compatible with most other drugs.

Charcoal acts by adsorbing gas bubbles by attracting them and adhering to them. It also adsorbs other medications, preventing them from being absorbed into the bloodstream. In fact, charcoal is used as a treatment for poisoning and medication overdose.

You can see how combining charcoal with your other medications may make them less effective (or even ineffective). Therefore, if you are taking other medications, it may be better to use simethicone instead of charcoal capsules for intestinal gas.

## DRUG INTERACTION CHART:
## MEDICATIONS TO TREAT DIARRHEA/
## CONSTIPATION/INTESTINAL GAS

| Drug Interaction | Rating* | Potential Effects/Recommendations |
|---|---|---|
| Charcoal/ Acetaminophen | C | See Key 35. |
| Charcoal/Barbiturates | C | See Key 22. |
| Charcoal/Depakene | A | See Key 30. |
| Charcoal/Diabetes Medicines | A | See Key 28. |
| Charcoal/Digoxin | A | See Key 17. |
| Charcoal/Dilantin | A | See Key 30. |
| Charcoal/Lasix | A | See Key 13. |
| Charcoal/Methotrexate | A | See Key 33. |
| Charcoal/Tegretol | A | See Key 30. |
| Charcoal/Tetracycline | A | See Key 31. |
| Charcoal/Theophylline | A | See Key 20. |
| Citrate of Magnesia/ Digoxin | D | See Key 17. |
| Citrate of Magnesia/ Tetracycline | A | See Key 31. |
| Kaopectate/Digoxin | C | See Key 17. |
| Kaopectate/ Phenothiazines | D | See Key 24. |
| Kaopectate/Quinidine | C | See Key 16. |
| Milk of Magnesia/ Digoxin | D | See Key 17. |
| Milk of Magnesia/ Tetracycline | A | See Key 31. |
| Mineral Oil/Vitamin A | D | See Key 41. |

| Drug Interaction | Rating* | Potential Effects/Recommendations |
|---|---|---|
| Pepto-Bismol/Anturane | A | See Key 26 . |
| Pepto-Bismol/Aspirin | C | See Key 35. |
| Pepto-Bismol/ Methotrexate | A | See Key 33. |
| Pepto-Bismol/ Salicylates | A | See Key 35. |
| Pepto-Bismol/ Tetracycline | A | See Key 31. |

* The rating indicates how harmful a drug interaction may be and how frequently it may occur.

"A" indicates a drug interaction that may cause serious harm and occurs frequently. "B" indicates a drug interaction that may cause serious harm but occurs less frequently. "C" indicates a drug interaction that is less harmful but occurs frequently. "D" indicates a drug interaction that is less harmful and occurs less frequently. See Key 9 for more information about the rating system.

# 38

# SLEEP AIDS

Nonprescription *sleep aids* are very different from sleeping pills that require a prescription. Sleep products such as Nytol and Sominex do not contain benzodiazepines or barbiturates (Keys 21 and 22), as do the prescription products. Instead, they contain medications that are members of the antihistamine category of drugs, such as diphenhydramine.

You may recognize diphenhydramine as the active ingredient in Benadryl. Yes, it is the same drug, but used for a different purpose. Diphenhydramine causes sleepiness, which is one of its most bothersome side effects when used as an allergy medication. In sleep aids this side effect is put to good use!

All three antihistamines used in sleep aids (doxylamine, pyrilamine, and diphenhydramine) tend to cause more sleepiness than the other antihistamines on the market. That is the reason why they were chosen as the active ingredient in many sleep aids.

## The Medications

Some nonprescription sleep aids are as follows:
1. diphenhydramine: *Compōz, Nervine, Nytol, Sleep-Eze 3, Sominex,* and *Twilite.*
2. doxylamine: *Unisom.*
3. pyrilamine: *Dormarex.*

One other sleep product, *Quiet World,* contains pyrilamine and small doses of acetaminophen and aspirin.

## Side Effects and Drug Interactions

The sleep-aid antihistamines are usually well-tolerated, although dry mouth may occur. The only problem with nonprescription sleep aids is that they may not be effective for some people, particularly those who awake in the early morning hours. In addition, some people feel stimulated by these antihistamines—and this is the last thing anyone wants from a sleeping pill!

Sleeplessness often increases with age; as people get older, they tend to need less sleep. However, if you are not sleeping well at night or feel tired the next morning, you may want to try one of the nonprescription sleep aids. If it does not work, perhaps your doctor will want to give you a prescription sleep aid.

If you do decide to try a nonprescription sleep aid, be careful not to combine it with other drug products that contain antihistamines. You may experience extreme sedation, dry mouth, blurred vision, and dizziness.

Because so many drug products contain antihistamines for different purposes, it is easy to inadvertently take two medications that contain antihistamines, thereby creating a drug-duplication type of interaction. If you look at the drug interaction chart for this Key, you will see examples of drug interactions that are really drug duplications. To avoid this problem, check with your pharmacist before combining any nonprescription medications.

### DRUG INTERACTION CHART: SLEEP AIDS

| Drug Interaction | Rating* | Potential Effects/Recommendations |
| --- | --- | --- |
| Sleep Aids (Nonprescription)/ Alcohol | A | You may experience excessive drowsiness, lack of coordination, and blurred vision. Do not take sleeping aids with alcoholic beverages. |
| Sleep Aids (Nonprescription)/ Antihistamines | A | *Drug duplication:* both medications are antihistamines, and they should not be taken together. |
| Sleep Aids (Nonprescription)/ Benylin Cough Syrup | A | *Drug duplication:* both medications are antihistamines, and they should not be taken together. |

| Drug Interaction | Rating* | Potential Effects/Recommendations |
|---|---|---|
| Sleep Aids (Nonprescription)/ Bonine Motion Sickness Tablets | A | *Drug duplication:* both medications are antihistamines, and they should not be taken together. |
| Sleep Aids (Nonprescription)/ Compazine | A | *Drug duplication:* both medications are antihistamines, and they should not be taken together. |
| Sleep Aids (Nonprescription)/ Dramamine | A | *Drug duplication:* both medications are antihistamines, and they should not be taken together. |
| Sleep Aids (Nonprescription)/ Phenothiazines | A | *Drug duplication:* both medications are antihistamines, and they should not be taken together. |
| Sleep Aids (Nonprescription)/ Phenergan | A | *Drug duplication:* both medications are antihistamines, and they should not be taken together. |
| Sleep Aids (Nonprescription)/ Thorazine | A | *Drug duplication:* both medications are antihistamines, and they should not be taken together. |

* The rating indicates how harmful a drug interaction may be and how frequently it may occur.

"A" indicates a drug interaction that may cause serious harm and occurs frequently. "B" indicates a drug interaction that may cause serious harm but occurs less frequently. "C" indicates a drug interaction that is less harmful but occurs frequently. "D" indicates a drug interaction that is less harmful and occurs less frequently. See Key 9 for more information about the rating system.

# 39

# COUGH MEDICINES

Cough medicines don't contain just cough medicine any more. Most cough products contain at least two or three active ingredients; some have four or five. Manufacturers have tried everything to make their products stand out from the rest. Recall the ad for Vick's NyQuil: "the nighttime sniffling, sneezing, coughing, aching, stuffy head, fever, so you can rest medicine."

What could be in that product to relieve all of those symptoms? Just one decongestant, one antihistamine, one cough suppressant, one pain reliever, and 25 percent alcohol (50 proof)! (Combining an antihistamine with alcohol *should* make you sleep!)

Is it better to take a cough medicine that provides all of the ingredients in one dose or to take the medications separately? As a pharmacist, I prefer cough medicines that do not contain pain relievers or alcohol. If you need a pain reliever, you can always take one separately in the dose that you desire. And nobody really needs that much alcohol.

Which cough medicine is the best one? The best one *for you* will depend on your symptoms and your medical condition. For example, if your nose and chest are congested and you are coughing, you want a cough medicine that contains a decongestant, an expectorant, and a cough suppressant. However, if you have high blood pressure, you should not take a cough medicine that contains a decongestant without first checking with your doctor because it may increase your blood pressure.

Cough medicines may contain one or more of the following ingredients:

1. cough suppressants, which stop unnecessary coughing.
2. expectorants, which thin mucus secretions in the bronchial airways.

3. antihistamines, which relieve itchy eyes and sneezing (see Key 40).
4. decongestants, which relieve nasal congestion (see Key 40).
5. pain relievers (see Key 35).
6. alcohol (not a medication).

There is a cough medicine for everyone's needs: sugar-free cough medicines are available for diabetics; alcohol-free cough medicines, for persons who cannot ingest alcohol or are taking medications that may interact with alcohol; and dye-free cough medicines, for those who have allergies to dyes commonly found in medicines.

## The Medications

Two types of nonprescription medications are used to treat cough:

1. cough suppressants: *dextromethorphan* and *diphenhydramine.*
2. expectorants: *guaifenesin*; others not proved to be effective but still used as expectorants are *ammonium chloride, sodium citrate,* and *terpin hydrate.*

## Side Effects and Drug Interactions

Dextromethorphan is usually well tolerated and is effective in reducing unnecessary coughing. It is often abbreviated as "DM" on the labels of cough medicines such as Robitussin DM. Compared to codeine, which is contained only in prescription cough products, dextromethorphan is thought to be just as effective. Unlike codeine, however, dextromethorphan does not cause such side effects as drowsiness, dizziness, and constipation.

Diphenhydramine is the cough suppressant in Benylin Cough Syrup. You may be familiar with diphenhydramine as the antihistamine in Benadryl liquid. In fact, diphenhydramine is probably the one nonprescription medication with the most uses. It serves as an antihistamine for allergies and allergic reactions, a cough suppressant, a sleep aid, and a motion sickness preventive. Used on the skin, it relieves itching caused by poison ivy and other minor skin irritations. For drug interactions involving diphenhydramine, see Key 40, "Antihistamines" or "Benadryl."

Guaifenesin, an expectorant, is usually well tolerated. To increase its effectiveness in loosening mucus secretions, drink plenty of water throughout the day. Using a humidifier or vaporizer also helps to thin mucus.

Drug interactions involving nonprescription cough medicines are usually due to the antihistamine or alcohol in the cough product. Cough medicines that contain high concentrations of alcohol such as NyQuil Nighttime Cold Medicine (25 percent alcohol), Contac Nighttime Cold Medicine (25 percent alcohol), and Terpin Hydrate Elixir (42 percent alcohol) may interact with other medications.

Before you purchase a cough medicine, have your pharmacist check it to ensure that you haven't selected a product that will interfere with other medications you are taking or with an existing medical condition.

## DRUG INTERACTION CHART:
## COUGH MEDICINES

| Drug Interaction | Rating* | Potential Effects/Recommendations |
|---|---|---|
| Benylin Cough Syrup/Benadryl | A | *Drug duplication:* the medications are the same drug, diphenhydramine. They should not be taken together. |
| Contac Nighttime Cold Medicine Liquid/Flagyl | A | This cough medicine has a high alcohol content (25 percent). If you combine it with Flagyl, you may experience nausea, facial flushing, dizziness, and blurred vision. |

| Drug Interaction | Rating* | Potential Effects/Recommendations |
|---|---|---|
| NyQuil Nighttime Cold Medicine Liquid/Flagyl | A | This cough medicine has a high alcohol content (25 percent). If you combine it with Flagyl, you may experience nausea, facial flushing, dizziness, and blurred vision. |
| Terpin Hydrate Elixir/Flagyl | A | This cough medicine has a high alcohol content (42 percent). If you combine it with Flagyl, you may experience nausea, facial flushing, dizziness, and blurred vision. |

* The rating indicates how harmful a drug interaction may be and how frequently it may occur.

"A" indicates a drug interaction that may cause serious harm and occurs frequently. "B" indicates a drug interaction that may cause serious harm but occurs less frequently. "C" indicates a drug interaction that is less harmful but occurs frequently. "D" indicates a drug interaction that is less harmful and occurs less frequently. See Key 9 for more information about the rating system.

# 40

## ALLERGY AND
## SINUS PRODUCTS

Both allergy and sinus drug products relieve nasal congestion; what, then, is the difference between them? Most allergy products contain an antihistamine and a decongestant; sinus medications usually contain a decongestant and a pain reliever.

Antihistamines relieve *allergy* and *common cold* symptoms, such as red, itchy, watery eyes, itchy nose, sneezing and nasal congestion. Decongestants relieve *nasal congestion*. Sometimes two different medications that work differently are needed to relieve congestion.

Antihistamines prevent the action of histamine, a natural body substance that dilates blood vessels in the nasal passages to cause congestion. In contrast, decongestants constrict nasal blood vessels that have already been dilated. In simple terms, antihistamines *prevent* congestion and decongestants *treat* congestion. Most allergy products contain both because the combination of an antihistamine and a decongestant is usually more effective than either medication used alone.

*Sinus products* contain a pain reliever for "sinus headaches" and a decongestant to reduce the congestion that may be causing the headache.

Most nasal sprays contain a decongestant that acts directly on the nasal passage to constrict dilated blood vessels. Some nasal sprays contain only saline (salt water) for those who cannot take decongestants. Although saline may not be as effective as a decongestant, it does provide relief.

### The Medications

Some of the nonprescription allergy and sinus products are as follows:

1. nonprescription antihistamines: *Actidil, Benadryl,*

*chlorpheniramine, Chlor-Trimeton, Dimetane, diphen-hydramine, Nolahist, pyrilamine,* and *Teldrin.*
2. nonprescription decongestants
   a. taken by mouth: *Afrinol, phenylpropanolamine (PPA), Propagest, pseudoephedrine, phenyleph-rine and Sudafed.*
   b. available as nasal spray or drops: *Afrin, Allerest 12-Hour Nasal, Coricidin Nasal Mist, Dristan Long Acting, Duration, Neo-Synephrine, Otrivin, NTZ Long Acting Nasal, Privine, Sinex Long Acting, Tyzine Drops,* and *4-Way Long Acting Nasal.*
3. saline nasal sprays: *Ocean Mist, NaSal Saline Nasal,* and *Salinex.*

Many of these medications are available in the timed-release dosage form as well as in the regular (immediate release) form.

Here are examples of some drug products that contain more than one ingredient:

## Allergy Drug Products

*Actifed* = Sudafed + triprolidine (antihistamine)
*Allerest Maximum Strength Tablets* = Sudafed + Chlor-Trimeton
*A. R. M. Caplets* = PPA + Chlor-Trimeton
*Benadryl Decongestant* = Benadryl + Sudafed
*Chlor-Trimeton Decongestant Tablets* = Chlor-Trimeton + Sudafed
*Demazin Tablets* = PPA + Chlor-Trimeton
*Dimetane Decongestant* = Dimetane + phenylephrine (decongestant)
*Dimetapp Extentabs* = PPA + Dimetane
*Sudafed Plus* = Sudafed + Chlor-Trimeton

## Sinus Products

*CoAdvil Caplets* = Sudafed + ibuprofen
*Contac Maximum Strength Sinus Caplets* = Sudafed + acetaminophen

*Maximum Strength Dristan Caplets* = Sudafed + acetaminophen

*Maximum Strength Sudafed Sinus Caplets* = Sudafed + acetaminophen

*Maximum Strength Tylenol Sinus Caplets* = Sudafed + acetaminophen

*Rhinocaps* = PPA + acetaminophen + aspirin

*Ursinus Inlay-Tabs* = Sudafed + aspirin

## Side Effects and Drug Interactions

### Antihistamines

The most common side effects of antihistamines are drowsiness and dizziness. In addition, they may reduce reaction time. This is an important fact to consider if you drive a car. For older people whose reflexes may not be as quick as they once were, reduced reaction time caused by an antihistamine may increase the risk of a traffic accident.

Therefore, if you are going on a car trip and plan to do some of the driving, ask your pharmacist to help you select a product that does not contain an antihistamine. If other nonprescription medications are not effective in relieving your allergy symptoms, talk to your doctor. Two prescription antihistamines (Hismanal and Seldane) that are less likely to cause drowsiness and dizziness, or affect your reaction time, are available.

Antihistamines are not only used for allergy. Some are used as nonprescription sleep aids, or are contained in pain relievers and in cough medicines. One antihistamine, diphenhydramine, is used for allergy, as a motion sickness preventive, as a sleep aid, and as a cough suppressant.

Because so many kinds of medications contain antihistamines, it is important to know what you are taking when you combine nonprescription medications. To avoid drug duplications (and the unwanted side effects that may result), ask your pharmacist to tell you what kinds of medications your nonprescription products contain. Write this information on a sheet of paper and keep it with your medications so that you can refer to it before taking two or more nonprescription medications together.

## Decongestants

Decongestants may cause nervousness, increased heart rate, and insomnia (if taken a few hours before bedtime). If you have high blood pressure, you may not be able to take decongestants because increased blood pressure may result. Check with your doctor before taking any oral product or nasal spray or drops that contain decongestants.

Beware of the drug interaction between decongestants and diet aids that contain phenylpropanolamine (PPA). This is a drug duplication.

### DRUG INTERACTION CHART: ALLERGY AND SINUS PRODUCTS

| Drug Interaction | Rating* | Potential Effects/Recommendations |
|---|---|---|
| Antihistamines/ Alcohol | A | See Key 43. |
| Antihistamines/ Antispasmodics | C | See Key 11. |
| Antihistamines/ Compazine | A | See Key 24 and Key 25, "Phenothiazines/Antihistamines." |
| Antihistamines/ Reglan | D | See Key 11. |
| Antihistamines/ Sleep Aids (Nonprescription) | A | See Key 38. |
| Antihistamines/ Sleep Medications | A | See Key 21. |
| Antihistamines/ Thorazine | A | See Key 24 and Key 25, "Phenothiazines/Antihistamines." |
| Antihistamines/ Transderm Scōp | A | See Key 25. |

| Drug Interaction | Rating* | Potential Effects/Recommendations |
|---|---|---|
| Benadryl/Benylin Cough Syrup | A | *Drug duplication:* both drug products contain the same medication, diphenhydramine. They should not be taken together. |
| Chlor-Trimeton/ Dilantin | D | See Key 30. |
| Decongestants/ Aldomet | A | See Key 12. |
| Decongestants/ Beta Blockers | B | See Key 14. |
| Decongestants/ Diet Aids (PPA) | A | *Drug duplication:* the medications are chemically similar and should not be taken together. |
| Decongestants/Ismelin | C | See Key 12. |
| Decongestants/MAOIs | A | See Key 23. |
| Decongestants/ Reserpine | B | See Key 12. |
| Decongestants/TCAs | A | See Key 23. |
| Neo-Synephrine Nasal Spray/Inderal | B | See Key 14. |
| Neo-Synephrine Nasal Spray/MAOIs | C | Neo-Synephrine may have a more potent effect. Ask your doctor whether you may use Neo-Synephrine while taking an MAOI. |
| Neo-Synephrine Nasal Spray/TCAs | B | See Key 23. |

* The rating indicates how harmful a drug interaction may be and how frequently it may occur.

"A" indicates a drug interaction that may cause serious harm and occurs frequently. "B" indicates a drug interaction that may cause serious harm but occurs less frequently. "C" indicates a drug interaction that is less harmful but occurs frequently. "D" indicates a drug interaction that is less harmful and occurs less frequently. See Key 9 for more information about the rating system.

# 41

## VITAMINS/MINERALS/ DIET AIDS/SALT SUBSTITUTES

People who take *vitamins*, go on *diets,* and use *salt substitutes* instead of table salt are generally regarded as healthy people who are taking good care of themselves. Rarely are these products associated with side effects, or recognized as medications that have the potential to interact with other medications.

However, as you glance at the drug interaction chart for this Key, you can see how many vitamins and minerals actually do interact with other medications. Moreover, some diet aids contain phenylpropanolamine (PPA), an ingredient also used as a decongestant in several nonprescription cold and allergy drug products. Taking diet aids that contain PPA with drug products that contain decongestants creates a drug duplication.

Most salt substitutes contain potassium chloride instead of table salt, which is sodium chloride. They are used mostly by people who must limit their sodium intake. Conditions that may require a salt-restricted diet are high blood pressure, congestive heart failure, and kidney disease.

### The Medications

The vitamins and minerals that may interact with other medications are as follows:

1. Vitamin A is a fat-soluble vitamin contained in cod-liver oil capsules and multivitamins.
2. Vitamin $B_6$, also referred to as "pyridoxine," is a water-soluble vitamin contained in B-complex and multivitamins.

185

3. Calcium is a mineral contained in *Caltrate*, *Os-cal*, some antacids such as *TUMS*, and dairy products such as milk, cheese, yogurt, and ice cream.
4. Iron, a mineral used to treat iron deficiency anemia, is available alone *(Femiron, Feosol, Fergon, Ferro-Sequels, ferrous sulfate, Mol-Iron, Slow FE)* and in multivitamins
5. Zinc, a mineral involved in many body functions, is available alone and in multivitamins.

Some nonprescription diet aids that contain PPA are *Acutrim, Appedrine, Dexatrim, Grapefruit Diet Plan with Diadax,* and *Prolamine*.

There are many brands of salt substitutes; the following contain potassium chloride: *Adolph's Salt Substitute, Morton Salt Substitute, NoSalt,* and *Nu-Salt*.

## Side Effects and Drug Interactions

### Vitamins and Minerals

Some vitamins, such as $B_6$, directly interfere with the action of other medications. Minerals such as calcium, iron, and zinc may bind to other medications, thereby preventing their absorption into the bloodstream; this may cause them to lose effectiveness.

### Diet Aids

The combination of diet aids and drug products that contain PPA represents a drug duplication which may cause you to feel excitable, nervous, and anxious. You may experience fast heart rate and insomnia. Ask your pharmacist to help you select allergy or cold products that will not interact with the diet aid you are using.

### Salt Substitutes

Salt substitutes contain potassium, an element that can interact with some diuretics that retain potassium. If you are taking a potassium-sparing diuretic such as Aldactone, amiloride, Dyrenium, Midamor, spironolactone, or triamterene, check with your doctor before using a salt substitute. If your doctor does allow this product, use the least amount that will improve the taste of your food. Avoid excessive amounts of salt substitutes; too much potassium in the bloodstream may lead to unwanted side effects.

## DRUG INTERACTION CHART: VITAMINS/MINERALS/DIET AIDS/ SALT SUBSTITUTES

| Drug Interaction | Rating* | Potential Effects/Recommendations |
|---|---|---|
| Calcium/CCBs | C | See Key 15. |
| Calcium/Tetracycline | A | See Key 31. |
| Calcium/Thiazides | B | This combination may lead to too much calcium in the bloodstream. Check with your doctor before taking calcium supplements. |
| Calcium/TUMS | A | *Drug duplication:* TUMS antacid contains the active ingredient calcium carbonate. If you are taking several doses of TUMS and calcium supplements every day, you may be getting too much calcium. Ask your pharmacist to help you determine the dosage of calcium that is safe for you. |
| Diet Aids (PPA)/ Aldomet | A | See Key 12. |
| Diet Aids (PPA)/ Ismelin | C | See Key 12. |
| Diet Aids (PPA)/ Decongestants | A | See Key 40. |
| Folic Acid/Dilantin | B | See Key 30. |
| Iron/Aldomet | C | See Key 12. |
| Iron/Antacids | C | Iron may be less effective. Take iron two hours before or four hours after the antacid. |
| Iron/Cipro | A | See Key 31. |

187

| Drug Interaction | Rating* | Potential Effects/Recommendations |
|---|---|---|
| Iron/Tagamet | D | Iron may be less effective. Take iron one hour before Tagamet. |
| Iron/Tetracycline | A | See Key 31. |
| Niacin/Mevacor | B | See Key 18. |
| Salt Substitutes/ Aldactone | B | See Key 13. |
| Vitamin A/Mineral Oil | D | Vitamin A may be less effective. Take vitamin A several hours before or after mineral oil. |
| Vitamin $B_6$/Dilantin | C | See Key 30. |
| Vitamin $B_6$/Levodopa | A | See Key 34. |
| Vitamin D/Thiazides | D | You may be at increased risk for developing a high blood level of calcium. If you are taking a thiazide diuretic, do not take vitamin D without first asking your doctor. |
| Vitamin E/ Anticoagulants | A | See Key 19. |
| Zinc/Cipro | C | See Key 31. |
| Zinc/Tetracycline | A | See Key 31. |

* The rating indicates how harmful a drug interaction may be and how frequently it may occur.

"A" indicates a drug interaction that may cause serious harm and occurs frequently. "B" indicates a drug interaction that may cause serious harm but occurs less frequently. "C" indicates a drug interaction that is less harmful but occurs frequently. "D" indicates a drug interaction that is less harmful and occurs less frequently. See Key 9 for more information about the rating system.

# 42

## MISCELLANEOUS NONPRESCRIPTION DRUG INTERACTIONS

In this Key, we will focus on four types of *nonprescription medications*: motion sickness medications, bronchial inhalers, medications for nighttime leg cramps, and medications that help you to stay awake.

### The Medications

Motion sickness medications are members of the antihistamine class of medications. They include *Bonine, diphenhydramine, Dramamine,* and *Marezine.* Bonine contains meclizine, the same active ingredient that is in the prescription motion sickness medication Antivert.

The medication in nonprescription bronchial inhalers is *epinephrine,* which is the same as adrenaline. Epinephrine opens airways to relieve wheezing and improve breathing. Two brands of bronchial inhalers included in the drug interaction chart in this Key are *Bronkaid Mist* and *Primatene Mist.* However, other brands, such as *AsthmaHaler, Bronitin Mist,* and *Medihaler-Epi,* also interact.

The medication to relieve nighttime leg cramps is *quinine.* Some brands of quinine are *Legatrin*, *Q-Vel*, and the generic *quinine sulfate.*

The active ingredient in medication to keep you awake is *caffeine.* Note the dosage of caffeine, given below, in each brand. Just for comparison, one cup of fresh-brewed coffee contains 100 to 150 mg of caffeine; a cup of tea has 60 to 75 mg.

*No-Doz* = 100 mg; *Tirend* = 100 mg; *Vivarin* = 200 mg
*Quick Pep* = 150 mg of caffeine + 300 mg of dextrose (sugar)

Due to limitation of space, only No-Doz and Vivarin are included in the drug interaction chart in this Key. You may use either of these brands to check in the chart for interactions involving another brand.

## Side Effects and Drug Interactions

### Motion Sickness Medications

With motion sickness medications, like most antihistamines, you may experience such side effects as drowsiness, dizziness, dry mouth, and blurred vision. Therefore you should use caution if you will be doing the driving on a trip.

If you take allergy medications, beware: Most allergy medications also contain antihistamines. Combining allergy drug products with motion sickness medications may create a drug duplication that can lead to unwanted side effects.

### Bronchial Inhalers

The most common side effects of epinephrine are nervousness, restlessness, dizziness, palpitations, and insomnia. These reactions are less likely to occur with inhalers than with oral asthma or COPD medications because most of the dose stays in the bronchi. However, if you use high or frequent dosages, some may be absorbed into the bloodstream.

Here is a typical situation that may arise: If you are taking a nonselective beta blocker such as Inderal and you find that you are having difficulty breathing, you may try to solve the problem yourself by using a nonprescription bronchial inhaler. What you should do instead is tell your doctor. Some people who are borderline asthmatics may experience asthma symptoms for the first time when they take beta blockers.

If you find that bronchoinhalers are not effective in relieving your symptoms, contact your doctor. There are many prescription medications that are very effective in relieving wheezing and other symptoms of asthma.

## Medications for Nighttime Leg Cramps

The one side effect of quinine that should concern you is ringing in the ears, which may be an indication that you've had too much. Other side effects that may occur are headache, dizziness, nausea, and visual disturbances.

Quinine does interact with digoxin, a heart medication and with Coumadin, an anticoagulant.

## Medications to Keep You Awake

The most common side effects of drug products that contain caffeine to keep you awake are nervousness, shaking, muscle twitching, irritability, stomach upset, and increased urination. Dizziness, palpitations, and rapid pulse may be an indication that you've had too much. If these symptoms occur, stop taking caffeine medications and also avoid foods and beverages that contain caffeine.

If you suffer from diabetes, angina pectoris, or other kinds of heart disease, it is a good idea to check with your doctor before taking a medication that contains caffeine. Caffeine has been linked to increased risk of heart disease and may also increase the risk of hyperglycemia in diabetics.

### DRUG INTERACTION CHART: MISCELLANEOUS NONPRESCRIPTION DRUG INTERACTIONS

| Drug Interaction | Rating* | Potential Effects/Recommendations |
| --- | --- | --- |
| Bonine/Antihistamines | A | *Drug duplication:* both medications are antihistamines, and they should not be taken together. |
| Bronkaid Mist/TCAs | B | Excessive inhalation of Bronkaid Mist may lead to increased blood pressure. Ask your doctor if you may use Bronkaid Mist with your TCA. |
| Dramamine/ Antihistamines | A | *Drug duplication:* both medications are antihistamines, and they should not be taken together. |

| Drug Interaction | Rating* | Potential Effects/Recommendations |
|---|---|---|
| No-Doz/Alcohol | — | No interaction! No-Doz will not reduce intoxication caused by alcohol consumption. |
| No-Doz/Cipro | D | No-Doz may have a more potent effect. |
| No-Doz/Tagamet | D | No-Doz may have a more potent effect. |
| Primatene Mist/TCAs | B | Excessive inhalation of Primatene Mist may lead to increased blood pressure. Ask your doctor whether you may use Primatene Mist with your TCA. |
| Quinine (in Q-Vel, Legatrin)/Coumadin | B | See Key 19. |
| Quinine (in Q-Vel, Legatrin)/Digoxin | B | See Key 17. |
| Vivarin/Alcohol | — | No interaction! Vivarin will not reduce intoxication caused by alcohol consumption. |
| Vivarin/Cipro | D | Vivarin may have a more potent effect. |
| Vivarin/Tagamet | D | Vivarin may have a more potent effect. |

* The rating indicates how harmful a drug interaction may be and how frequently it may occur.

"A" indicates a drug interaction that may cause serious harm and occurs frequently. "B" indicates a drug interaction that may cause serious harm but occurs less frequently. "C" indicates a drug interaction that is less harmful but occurs frequently. "D" indicates a drug interaction that is less harmful and occurs less frequently. See Key 9 for more information about the rating system.

192

# 43

## ALCOHOL AND DRUGS THAT DO NOT MIX

We are all aware of how *alcoholic beverages* (ethanol) affect our senses. However, most people would not classify them as drugs. Some people include beer or wine, like soda pop, in their daily diets and may unknowingly combine their medication with these alcoholic beverages. The result may be unwanted and unexpected side effects.

### Effect of Ethanol on the Central Nervous System

Ethanol itself *is* a drug and may produce a potent effect on the central nervous system (CNS), the so-called "switchboard" of the body. At first, intoxication with ethanol may produce effects such as giddiness, dizziness, and a feeling of euphoria. As intoxication progresses, however, other effects—drowsiness, loss of coordination, blurred vision, slurred speech, nausea, and vomiting—may occur.

Most people act responsibly when it comes to medications and alcoholic beverages. They know how they react to their medications and to alcohol, and they try not to overdo. However, some people may be in for a big surprise if they attempt to take their medication (or forgot that they took it) and have "just a *few* drinks." The reaction—extreme sleepiness, stupor, and perhaps loss of consciousness—may be overwhelming.

Often, people do not understand why a reaction like this may occur from the combination of medications and alcohol. The reason is that the combined action of the two is much more powerful than the action of the medication or the alcoholic beverage alone. To simplify this point, here $1 + 1 = 3$ instead of what you would normally expect: $1 + 1 = 2$.

# Other Kinds of Alcohol/Drug Interactions

Alcohol may interact with aspirin and with acetaminophen to produce rare but harmful side effects. Aspirin and alcohol can each irritate the gastrointestinal lining. Together, they may cause bleeding in some people.

Both alcohol and acetaminophen may cause damage to the liver if taken every day over several weeks or months. Combining the recommended dosage of acetaminophen and one alcoholic drink once in a while is less likely to have an effect on the liver.

Some medications, such as Antabuse, Diabinese (chlorpropamide), and Flagyl, may interact with alcohol and induce the *disulfiram reaction*, which causes severe nausea and vomiting, throbbing headache, sweating, and facial flushing. Do not drink alcoholic beverages when you are taking any of these medications.

Finally, there is one "nondrug interaction" I would like to emphasize. It involves alcohol and coffee. Very often, people who are already intoxicated remember that they have to drive home. They believe that caffeinated coffee will reverse the intoxicating effects of alcohol. However, *this is not true!* Therefore, you should not assume that the caffeine will "take effect" anytime soon, and you should not drive.

There is one common belief that is true, however. You are less likely to become intoxicated if you drink an alcoholic beverage with a meal or on a full stomach, as compared to doing so without food.

# DRUG INTERACTION CHART:
## ALCOHOL AND DRUGS THAT DO NOT MIX

| Drug Interaction | Rating* | Potential Effects/Recommendations |
|---|---|---|
| Alcohol/ Acetaminophen | C | See Key 35. |
| Alcohol/ Anticoagulants | D | See Key 19. |
| Alcohol/ Antihistamines | A | You may experience excessive drowsiness and lack of coordination. It is best to avoid this combination. |
| Alcohol/Aspirin | B | See Key 35. |
| Alcohol/Barbiturates | A | See Key 22. |
| Alcohol/ Benzodiazepines | A | See Key 21. |
| Alcohol/CCBs | A | See Key 15. |
| Alcohol/Diabetes Medicines | A | See Key 28. |
| Alcohol/Dilantin | C | See Key 30. |
| Alcohol/Flagyl | A | See Key 31. |
| Alcohol/Food | C | You may become less intoxicated by ingesting alcohol after eating a meal or drinking milk. It is best not to drink alcoholic beverages on an empty stomach. |
| Alcohol/Insulin | A | See Key 28. |
| Alcohol/Isoniazid (INH) | C | See Key 32. |
| Alcohol/MAOIs | A | See Key 23. |
| Alcohol/Meprobamate | A | See Key 21. |
| Alcohol/Methotrexate | D | See Key 33. |
| Alcohol/Mysoline | A | See Key 22. |
| Alcohol/Narcotic Pain Relievers | A | See Key 26. |
| Alcohol/Nitrates | A | See Key 15. |
| Alcohol/Nizoral | C | See Key 32. |
| Alcohol/Noctec | A | See Key 21. |
| Alcohol/Parlodel | B | See Key 34. |
| Alcohol/Phenothiazines | A | See Key 24. |

| Drug Interaction | Rating* | Potential Effects/Recommendations |
|---|---|---|
| Alcohol/Reglan | B | You may become intoxicated more quickly and to a greater degree. |
| Alcohol/Sleep Aids (Nonprescription) | A | See Key 38. |
| Alcohol/Tagamet | C | You may become intoxicated more quickly and to a greater degree. |
| Alcohol/TCAs | A | You may become intoxicated more quickly and to a greater degree. |
| Alcohol/ Transderm Scōp | A | See Key 25. |

* The rating indicates how harmful a drug interaction may be and how frequently it may occur.

"A" indicates a drug interaction that may cause serious harm and occurs frequently. "B" indicates a drug interaction that may cause serious harm but occurs less frequently. "C" indicates a drug interaction that is less harmful but occurs frequently. "D" indicates a drug interaction that is less harmful and occurs less frequently. See Key 9 for more information about the rating system.

# 44

# FOODS THAT INTERACT WITH DRUGS

You may be wondering why food interacts with some medications, but not with others. There are two main reasons.

### Interference with Absorption

One reason involves the absorption of medications into the bloodstream. If they are not completely absorbed, they may lose effectiveness.

The ease with which a medication is absorbed has to do mostly with the medication itself. Some drugs require certain conditions to dissolve, disintegrate, and be absorbed. Here are some of the ways that food may interfere with the absorption of certain medications, and the steps you can take to prevent or minimize this effect:

1. *penicillin:* Penicillin is destroyed in the presence of acid, which is secreted in the stomach whenever we eat (or even smell food!)
   *Take penicillin on an empty stomach.*
2. *tetracycline:* Tetracycline binds with the calcium in milk and other dairy products and forms a complex. The complex cannot be absorbed through the gastrointestinal tract.
   *Take tetracycline at least one hour before or two hours after dairy products.*
3. *Hismanal:* Taken with food, Hismanal may lose up to 60% of its availability in the bloodstream.
   *Take Hismanal on an empty stomach.*
4. Some *theophylline* products: In this case, food does not appear to interfere with the drug itself, but rather with the type of dosage form it is contained in (capsule,

197

tablet). Some brands of theophylline are better absorbed with a high-fat meal; others are less well absorbed. Still others are not affected.

*Take these theophylline products on an empty stomach or with a light snack, but not with a heavy meal.*

## Chemical Interference

The other principal reason why foods interfere with some medications is that these foods contain an ingredient that acts chemically with the medications. The best example is the interaction between monoamine oxidase inhibitors (MAOIs) and the many foods that contain tyramine, an amino acid. Combined, tyramine and MAOIs may cause a serious reaction in which blood pressure increases suddenly. Fatalities have occurred with MAOI/tyramine interactions.

Here is a list of some foods with a high tyramine content:

1. cheeses: Boursault, Camembert, Cheddar, Gruyere, and Stilton.
2. meats and fish: balogna, herring (dried or pickled), pepperoni, salami, summer sausage, and any other fermented or spoiled meat.
3. marmite (a yeast extract).

The following foods have a moderate to low tyramine content:

1. cheeses: American, blue, Brie, mozzarella, Parmesan, Romano, and Roquefort.
2. yogurt and sour cream.
3. meats and fish: chicken liver and caviar.
4. overripe fruits and vegetables: avocados, bananas, bean curd, canned figs, miso soup, raisins, and soy sauce.
5. alcoholic beverages: beer, Chianti and other red wines, and sherry.
6. seasoning: meat tenderizer.

Broad beans (fava beans) do not contain tyramine, but do have another ingredient that may produce the same reaction as tyramine when combined with MAOIs.

If you are taking a MOAI, you should avoid these foods. An easy way to remember what not to eat is to avoid aged or overripe foods, fermented or spoiled meats, and red wines.

## DRUG INTERACTION CHART:
## FOODS THAT INTERACT WITH DRUGS

| Drug Interaction | Rating* | Potential Effects/Recommendations |
|---|---|---|
| Food/Alcohol | C | See Key 43. |
| Food/Anticoagulants | C | See Key 19. |
| Food/Beta Blockers | C | See Key 14 |
| Food/Calan SR | C | See Key 15. |
| Food/Capoten | C | See Key 12. |
| Food/Carafate | A | See Key 10. |
| Food/Fulvicin | C | See Key 32. |
| Food/Hismanal | A | See Key 27. |
| Food/Isoniazid (INH) | C | See Key 32. |
| Food/Macrodantin | C | See Key 31. |
| Food/MAOIs | B | See Key 23. |
| Food/Mevacor | C | See Key 18. |
| Food/Noroxin | A | See Key 31. |
| Food/Penicillin | A | See Key 31. |
| Food/Questran | A | See Key 18. |
| Food/Tetracycline | A | See Key 31. |
| Food/Theophylline | C | See Key 20. |
| Salt (Sodium Chloride)/ Lithium | C | See Key 24. |

* The rating indicates how harmful a drug interaction may be and how frequently it may occur.

"A" indicates a drug interaction that may cause serious harm and occurs frequently. "B" indicates a drug interaction that may cause serious harm but occurs less frequently. "C" indicates a drug interaction that is less harmful but occurs frequently. "D" indicates a drug interaction that is less harmful and occurs less frequently. See Key 9 for more information about the rating system.

# 45

## FIVE WAYS TO PREVENT DRUG INTERACTIONS

1. *If possible, purchase all of your prescription medications from one pharmacy.* This precaution is especially important if more than one doctor prescribes medication for you. Most doctors keep a record of the medications they prescribe, but they do not keep a record of medications that other doctors prescribe. If you have all of your prescriptions filled at one pharmacy, the pharmacist can easily detect potential drug interactions between medications that different doctors have prescribed.

   In addition, your pharmacist can make sure that your new prescription medication does not interact with any prescription you had filled in the past. Many people refuse to throw away old prescription medications, even if they are not taking them any longer. Your pharmacist can alert you not to combine the new medication with another that you may have at home.

2. *If you cannot purchase all of your prescription medications from one pharmacy, ask your doctor to check all of your medications, including the ones prescribed by different doctors, for interactions.* Many people stay at their vacation homes for months at a time and need to have their prescriptions filled at a pharmacy nearby. This means that the pharmacy they use at home will not have a complete record of the medications they are taking. If you cannot use one pharmacy consistently, you may want to ask your doctor to check all of your medications, including, for example, the ones prescribed by your heart specialist and dentist, for interactions.

But beware; many doctors won't enjoy this task because it is time consuming.

3. *Keep a list of the medications you are currently using with you at all times.* Aside from the convenience of having available the names and doses of your medications at any time, your "Medication List" will provide critical information to health professionals if you are in an accident or need immediate medical treatment in a hospital emergency room.

Your list should include the name, strength, and dosing schedule for each medication. Remember to include nonprescription drug products in your list; many of these products contain several active ingredients that have the potential to interact with other drugs.

4. *Before you purchase a nonprescription drug product, ask your pharmacist if it is safe to combine the nonprescription drug with the drugs on your medication list.* Many of the drug products on the market today contain two, three, or even more active ingredients. In addition, some of these active ingredients can be found in several products that are unrelated. For example, diphenhydramine, an antihistamine, is the active ingredient in Benylin, a cough syrup, and in Nytol, a nonprescription sleep aid. Diphenhydramine is also one of the active ingredients in Benadryl Plus, a sinus/allergy preparation, and is commonly recommended to prevent allergic swelling reactions caused by bee stings. Taking two of these drug products at the same time could cause a potential overdose and serious side effects, especially if prescription drugs are also combined.

It is not uncommon for consumers to choose two nonprescription drugs that interact with each other or contain the same ingredient. Your list will help the pharmacist determine whether the drug product you are about to purchase will interact with other medications you have at home.

5. *Most important, keep your checkup appointments with your doctor*. Only your doctor can make sure that your drug therapy is safe and effective for you. Because of the great variation in the way people react to medications, you must be examined by your doctor regularly. Do not assume that you will be taking the same dosages of the same medications for the rest of your life—your body changes as you grow older, and your doctor may have to adjust one or more of your medications from time to time. Although it may be frustrating (and expensive) to keep visiting your doctor when you feel well, these checkups can prevent serious medical problems that could result from the medications you are taking or your underlying medical condition.

# 46

## WHEN A NEW MEDICATION IS PRESCRIBED FOR YOU

What is the first thing that runs through your mind when you receive a prescription for a new medication from your doctor? If you are like most people, your first concern may be the possible side effects or the cost of the medication. But these are not the only questions you should have in mind.

Your first priority should be to learn all about your new medication and to know how to take it correctly. Keep in mind that if you take the medication exactly as your doctor and pharmacist have instructed, it is less likely that you will suffer side effects from it. Also, the cost of your medical care will most likely be less than for somebody who does *not* take his medication correctly; people who do not follow their drug treatment program generally end up seeing the doctor more often and switching medications—all which may cost more in the long run.

To learn about a new medication easily and quickly, use the list of questions below when your doctor prescribes the medication for you. Also, when you are getting a new prescription filled at your pharmacy for the first time, try to pick the medication up yourself. Your pharmacist can then review with you the proper way to take it and can also warn you if your other medications may interact with the new one.

Here are the questions you should ask your doctor or pharmacist before taking a new medication:

1. What is the name and strength of the medication?
2. Which medical condition is the medication for?
   If you are taking medications for two different medical conditions such as diabetes and high blood pres-

sure, make sure you know for which condition the new medication is being prescribed.

3. How should I take the medication?
   how many times a day?
   with or without food?
   any particular time in the day?
   take it until it is finished, or just until my symptoms are gone?

4. What are the common side effects of the medication?

5. Does the medication interact with other nonprescription drug products that I have at home?

6. Is it safe to drink alcoholic beverages with the medication?

7. What should I do if I miss a dose?

8. How should the medication be stored?
   in the refrigerator?
   protected from light?

9. Is a generic brand of the medication available? If so, is there a difference in cost in the generic and brand-name products?

10. Can my prescription be refilled? If so, how many times?

If you can answer these questions before you start taking your new medication, you've done your job as an informed patient and consumer. You have played an important role in your medication therapy and will most likely reap the benefit—better health. Remember: you should never hesitate to ask questions about your medications. As a pharmacist, I believe that your questions are important, and answering them to improve your drug therapy is the most satisfying part of my job!

# QUESTIONS AND ANSWERS

**Q. If you read in this book that two of the medications you are taking interact, should you stop taking (a) one of the medications or (b) both?**

A. Neither answer is correct! You should not change your medication therapy at all. Many drugs that interact with each other may be combined under certain circumstances. For example, some drugs that interact may be taken together as long as you are being checked regularly by your doctor via physical examinations or by lab tests.

If you are concerned about the effects of your medications when they are combined, speak to your doctor or pharmacist. Using professional knowledge and judgment, he or she will be able to evaluate your particular situation and answer your questions.

**Q. If a medication is known to cause serious side effects, should you not take it?**

A. The answer to this question depends on your illness. If your illness is more serious than the side effects of the medication, you are more likely to benefit from using the medication, despite the side effects, than from not taking it. On the other hand, if your illness is not serious and the side effects of the medication may cause considerable harm, taking the medication may not be worth the risk.

These two examples represent extreme cases. Usually, the benefit-to-risk factor is not clear-cut and requires your doctor's professional judgment.

Perhaps the following advice seems trivial, but it may prevent serious consequences: *Don't try to second-guess your doctor's judgment on the basis of what you've read in various books and magazine articles.* Keep in mind that nonprofessional literature is written to provide general information—to make you more aware of the questions you should ask your doctor. Only your doctor knows your particular situation and can make a sound decision, based on his training and experience, regarding your drug therapy.

**Q. My husband and I both suffer from high blood pressure and we both take the same medication. Our doctor told us that my husband may take a decongestant but that I may not. Why is this?**

A. Situations like this one happen quite often. One person may not be affected by a drug interaction, whereas another person may experience a pronounced effect. Because everyone's body makeup is different, the reaction to a particular medication or combination of medications is likely to vary from person to person.

**Q. Can all drug interactions be prevented by taking the medications several hours apart from each other?**

A. Not necessarily. Taking your medication dosages several hours apart from each other may work for some interactions in which drug absorption is hampered. Other kinds of drug interactions, however, cannot be prevented by separating the doses. Check the drug interaction charts in the various Keys of this book to see whether your medications should be taken several hours apart from each other.

**Q. Some of the drug names in this book start with an uppercase letter and others do not. Why is this?**

A. A drug name that starts with an uppercase letter represents the brand-name product of that medication. A drug name that begins with a lowercase letter is the generic name of the medication. For example, ibuprofen is the generic name; Advil is the brand name.

# GLOSSARY

**Absorption**   the passage of food and medications through the cells of the intestinal tract into the bloodstream.

**Adsorption**   the adhesion of one medication to another medication in the intestinal tract. When adsorbed, a medication is not "free" to pass through the intestinal tract into the bloodstream and will remain inactive.

**Blood level**   a measurement of the amount (concentration) of medication in the bloodstream. Doctors often use this measurement to tailor the dosage of a medication to the needs of each patient.

**Drug binding**   two medications (in the intestinal tract) that attach to each other in such a way that they form a new complex that cannot be absorbed into the bloodstream.

**Metabolism**   the breakdown of medications or foods into their byproducts. Some medications are metabolized into inactive byproducts before they are eliminated from the body.

**Potent**   1. a medication that requires very little of the active ingredient to produce its effect.

2. "a more potent effect"—the medication may produce a stronger effect than expected, which may result in unwanted side effects.

**Protein binding**   a medication that attaches itself to proteins in the bloodstream, and is therefore not "free" to produce its effects.

**Prothrombin time (PT)**   1. a test performed to determine if the blood is clotting properly.

2. a measurement of the length of time needed for blood to clot. The results may be used by doctors to adjust the dosage of anticoagulants.

**Receptor site**   the site (or specific area) in the body at which a medication produces its action.

**Secreted (or secretion)**   the discharge of a substance from a gland or organ (such as insulin from the pancreas).

# GENERIC/BRAND NAME INDEX

Most medications are best known by their brand names and are listed by brand name in this book. However, some medications are also well known by their generic names. If your medication is generic, this chart will help you find its brand name—which is the name you should use when you examine the drug interactions in the appropriate Keys.

| Generic Name | Brand Name | Generic Name | Brand Name |
|---|---|---|---|
| acetaminophen | Tylenol and others | ibuprofen | Motrin, Advil, Medipren, Motrin IB, Nuprin |
| allopurinol | Zyloprim | | |
| amantadine | Symmetrel | | |
| amiloride | Midamor | | |
| amitriptyline | Elavil | imipramine | Tofranil |
| benztropine | Cogentin | indomethacin | Indocin |
| carbamazepine | Tegretol | isosorbide dinitrate | Isordil |
| carisoprodol | Soma | lorazepam | Ativan |
| cephalexin | Keflex | meclizine | Antivert |
| chlordiazepoxide | Librium or Libritabs | methocarbamol | Robaxin |
| | | methyldopa | Aldomet |
| chlorpheniramine | Chlor-Trimeton | methylprednisolone | Medrol |
| chlorpromazine | Thorazine | metoclopramide | Reglan |
| chlorpropamide | Diabinese | metronidazole | Flagyl |
| chlorthalidone | Hygroton | nifedipine | Procardia or Adalat |
| chlorothiazide | Diuril | | |
| conjugated estrogens | Premarin | nortriptyline | Pamelor or Aventyl |
| cyclobenzaprine | Flexeril | | |
| desipramine | Norpramin | oxazepam | Serax |
| dexamethasone | Decadron | prazosin | Minipress |
| diazepam | Valium | prochlorperazine | Compazine |
| dicyclomine | Bentyl | procainamide | Procan or Pronestyl |
| digoxin* | Lanoxin | | |
| diphenhydramine | Benadryl | promethazine | Phenergan |
| disopyramide | Norpace | propranolol | Inderal |
| docusate sodium | Colace | pseudoephedrine | Sudafed |
| doxepin | Sinequan or Adapin | spironalactone | Aldactone |
| | | temazepam | Restoril |
| flurazepam | Dalmane | TMP-SMZ | Septra or Bactrim |
| furosemide | Lasix | triamterene | Dyrenium |
| haloperidol | Haldol | trihexyphenidyl | Artane |
| hydrochlorothiazide | Hydrodiuril or Esidrex | verapamil | Calan or Isoptin |

* Use *digoxin* instead of *Lanoxin* to look up your drug interactions.

# INDEX

(Generic drug names are *italicized*.)

209

210

211

212

213

214